PROLO YOUR PAIN AWAY!

PROLO YOUR PAIN AWAY!

Curing Chronic Pain With Prolotherapy

ROSS A. HAUSER, M.D. *Physical Medicine and Rehabilitation Specialist*

WITH *Marion A. Hauser, M.S., R.D., and Kurt Pottinger*

BEULAH LAND PRESS • OAK PARK, ILLINOIS

PROLO YOUR PAIN AWAY!

ISBN 0-9661010-0-6

© 1998, Beulah Land Press
Cover and page design by Kipland Publishing House
Illustrations by Megan H. Barnard, Chris Athens, Thomas Penna, and Joe Faraci

Published by Beulah Land Press
715 Lake Street, Suite 600, Oak Park, Illinois 60301

Printed in the United States of America
First Printing, January 1998
Second Printing, October 1998

CONTENTS

DISCLAIMER

The information presented in this book is based on the experiences of Gustav A. Hemwall, M.D., and Ross A. Hauser, M.D., and is intended for informational and educational purposes only. In no way should this book be used as a substitute for your own physician's advice.

Physicians should use and apply the technique of Prolotherapy only after they have received extensive training and demonstrated the ability to safely administer the treatment. The author, publisher, and publishing agent are not responsible if physicians who are unqualified in the use of Prolotherapy administer the treatment based solely on the contents of this book.

If Prolotherapy or any other treatment regime described in this book appear to apply to your condition, the author recommends that a formal evaluation be performed by a physician who is competent in treating chronic pain with Prolotherapy. Those desiring treatment should make medical decisions with the aid of a personal physician. No medical decisions should be made based solely on the contents or recommendations made in this book.

ACKNOWLEDGEMENTS

L ife has been good to me. I have enjoyed the support of parents who always told me to "just do my best," and the love of a wonderful family, especially that of my sister, Staci, my grandparents, and my in-laws.

A pupil is only as wise as his teachers. I have had wonderful teachers. Of course, none of my work in Prolotherapy would have been possible without the confidence placed in me by Gustav A. Hemwall, M.D. Thank you, Dr. Hemwall, for sharing what it means to be an "old-fashioned" doctor.

I would also like to thank my colleagues who have taught me many things: Jean Liu; Gail Gelsinger, R.N.; Harold J. Kristal, D.D.S.; Mike and Sue Aberle; Gary Martin, Ph.D.; Doug Kaufmann; Robert O'Hara, M.D.; Jay Subbarao, M.D., and staff at the Edward Hines Jr. V.A. Hospital; William Mauer, D.O.; and Paul Dommers, D.O.

I owe a great debt to Steven Elsasser, M.D., for taking me under his wing and showing me that "true medicine comes from the earth, not from a drug representative."

I am who I am partly because of my pastor, the late Peter Blakemore. Thank you, Pastor Peter, for showing me that true love comes only from God. I look forward to seeing you and Pastor John, Larry, Dr. Steve, and Dr. Dave when God calls me home.

What would anyone do without friends? I have been blessed with the greatest friends in the world: Don and Kristy; Marla and the kids; Tim, Sheila, and the kids; Steve and Candace; Mark and Janice; and the whole clan at Harrison Street Bible Church. They love me just the way I am, faults and all. To my friends in the old Thursday night Bible study group: Thank you for allowing me to be honest and for teaching me honesty.

Thank you, Bill, for helping us keep our business afloat. (He's our accountant and one of my high school buddies.)

What would the doctor do without the greatest staff in the world? To Kurt, Patsy, Marion, Nick, John, David, Jennifer, Bill, Lisa, Liz (my sister-in-law), Marylou, Alta, Peter, Mary, Chris, and Diana: Thank you for making work so enjoyable. Thank you for working so hard and lending a listening ear to those who have walked through our doors with hurts and sorrows.

I especially want to thank my wife, Marion, and Kurt, my business manager, for the many hours they spent editing this book. Books cannot be written without patience. A job well done! When can we start on the next one?!

Thank you to Joe Faraci for providing all of the initial illustrations and to Chris Athens, Megan Barnard, and Thomas Penna for completing them. A special thank you to the staff at Kipland Publishing House for putting up with this first-time author's idiosyncrasies. Thanks a million Cathy, Tonya, and K.J. I hope this book doesn't put us both under.

I also want to thank the many volunteers who give their time to Beulah Land Natural Medicine Clinic, especially Daphene Huffman; Mary Ellen Schlamer; Pastor Carl and Linda Fisher; Rodney Van Pelt, M.D.; Eddie Bennett; Kurt Ehling, D.C.; Dick Boomer (my father-in-law); Andrew and Peter Blakemore; Sheila, Heather, Heidi, Tim, and Toby Phillips; Brenda Lewis; and the rest of the wonderful volunteers from the First Baptist Church in Thebes, Harrison Street Bible Church in Oak Park, and the folks from southern Illinois and southeast Missouri.

Most of all, I would like to thank my wife and best friend who stays by my side no matter what fiasco I get us into. Thank you, Marion, for teaching me what goodness is all about. Thank you for giving up your career to help me run our clinic.

Finally, I want to say thank you to the One who makes it all possible. I agree with the words King David wrote several thousand years ago: "But as for me, I will always have hope; I will praise you more and more. My mouth will tell of your righteousness, of your salvation all day long, though I know not its measure. I will come and proclaim your mighty acts, O Sovereign LORD; I will proclaim your righteousness, yours alone."[1]

I wish everyone who reads this the best of health — but most importantly that you Prolo Your Pain Away!!

Sincerely with warm regards,

Ross A. Hauser M.D.

DEDICATION

This book is dedicated to God, who created the marvelous wonder we call the human body. Thank You, God, for giving us pain so we would know when something is wrong with the body You gave us. Thank You for allowing us to help the body heal. We acknowledge that all true healing comes from You.

"Jesus replied, 'Go back and report to John what you hear and see: The blind receive sight, the lame walk, those who have leprosy are cured, the deaf hear, the dead are raised, and the good news is preached to the poor.'"[1]

This book is also dedicated to two of God's faithful servants: Gustav and Helen Hemwall. They have traveled across the United States and to many countries helping orphans, the poor, and the destitute.

Many could testify that the "you" Jesus referred to in the following passage could be substituted with Gustav and Helen Hemwall. "Then the King will say to those on his right, 'Come, you who are blessed by my Father; take your inheritance, the kingdom prepared for you since the creation of the world. For I was hungry and you gave me something to eat, I was thirsty and you gave me something to drink, I was a stranger and you invited me in, I needed clothes and you clothed me, I was sick and you looked after me, I was in prison and you came to visit me.' Then the righteous will answer him, 'LORD, when did we see you hungry and feed you, or thirsty and give you something to drink? When did we see you a stranger and invite you in, or needing clothes and clothe you? When did we see you sick or in prison and go to visit you?' The King will reply, 'I tell you the truth, whatever you did for one of the least of these brothers of mine, you did for me.'"[2]

I would also like to dedicate this book to the late David Brewer, M.D., a good friend and former colleague who, through his excellent knowledge and skills, gave life to many people. Dr. Brewer was an inspiration to all in the medical profession, showing us how to love God and others. Many will truly miss you.

FOREWORD

The purpose of this book is to present Prolotherapy to the lay person in a comprehensive, yet readable language. Dr. Hauser has written this in a jocular fashion. He has covered every phase of Prolotherapy with definitions, explanations, and illustrations of the many problems of acute and chronic musculoskeletal pain.

Most of the writing is in simple lay language, but is intermingled with scientific terms. A person may not want to read the entire book, but select areas of pain that are of greatest interest. There are numerous references, so further study can be done if desired. Although the primary focus is on Prolotherapy, many alternative procedures are described.

The basic principle of the book is simplicity with emphasis on the most conservative methods of pain management. The various accounts of patients and the many examples given are all accurate and can be duplicated if the basic principles of Prolotherapy are followed.

G A Hemwall

Gustav A. Hemwall, M.D.
The world's most experienced Prolotherapist

A Word From C. Everett Koop, M.D.

Prolotherapy is the name some people use for a type of medical intervention in musculoskeletal pain that causes a proliferation of collagen fibers such as those found in ligaments and tendons, as well as a shortening of those fibers. The "prolo" in Prolotherapy, therefore, comes from proliferative.

Other therapists have referred to this type of treatment as Sclerotherapy. "Sclera" comes from the Greek word "sklera," which means hard. Sclerotherapy, therefore, refers to the same type of medical intervention which produces a hardening of the tissues treated—just as described above in the proliferation of collagen fibers.

Not many physicians are aware of Prolotherapy, and even fewer are adept at this form of treatment. One wonders why that is so. In my opinion, it is because medical folks are skeptical and Prolotherapy, unless you have tried it and proven its worth, seems to be too easy a solution to a series of complicated problems that afflict the human body and have been notoriously difficult to treat by any other method. Another reason is the simplicity of the therapy: Injecting an irritant solution, which may be something as simple as glucose, at the junction of a ligament with a bone to produce the rather dramatic therapeutic benefits that follow. Another very practical reason is that many insurance companies do not pay for Prolotherapy, largely because their medical advisors do not understand it, have not practiced it, and there-fore do not recommend it. Finally, Prolotherapy seems too simple a procedure for a very complicated series of musculoskeletal problems which affect huge numbers of patients. The reason why I consented to write the preface to this book is because I have been a patient who has benefitted from Prolotherapy. Having been so remark-ably relieved of my chronic disabling pain, I began to use it on some of my patients—but more on that later.

When I was 40 years old, I was diagnosed in two separate neurological clinics as having intractable (incurable) pain. My comment was that I was too young to have intractable pain. It was by chance that I learned that Gustav A. Hemwall, M.D., a practitioner in the suburbs of Chicago, was an expert in Prolotherapy. When I asked him if he could cure my pain, he asked me to describe it. When I had done the best that I could, he replied, "There is no such pain. Do you mean a pain...." And then he continued to describe my pain much better than I could. When I said, "That's it exactly," he said, "I can fix you." To make a long story short, my intractable pain was not intractable and I was remarkably improved to the point where my pain ceased to be a problem. Much milder recurrences of that pain over the next 20 years were retreated the same way with equally beneficial results.

I was so impressed with what Dr. Hemwall had done for me that on several occasions, just to satisfy my curiosity, I watched him work in his clinic and witnessed the unbelievable variety of musculoskeletal problems he was able to treat successfully. Many of his patients were people who had been treated for years by all sorts of methods, including major surgery, some of which had left them worse off than they were before. Many of his patients had the lack of confidence in further treatment and the low expectations that folks inflicted with chronic pain frequently exhibit. Yet I saw so many of them cured that I could not help but become a "believer" in Prolotherapy.

I was a pediatric surgeon, and there are not many times when Prolotherapy is needed in children because they just don't suffer from the same relaxation of musculoskeletal connections that are so amenable to treatment by Prolotherapy. But I noticed frequently that the parents of my patients were having difficulty getting into their coats, or they walked with a limp, or they favored an arm. I would ask what the problem was and then, if it seemed suitable, offer my services in Prolotherapy at no expense, feeling that I was a pediatric surgeon and this was really not my line of work. The results I saw in those many patients were just as remarkable as was the relief I had received in the hands of Dr. Hemwall. I was so impressed with what Prolotherapy could do for musculoskeletal disease that I, at one time, thought that might be the way I would spend my years after formal retirement from the University of Pennsylvania. But the call of President Reagan to be Surgeon General of the United States interrupted any such plans.

The reader may wonder why, in spite of what I have said and what this book contains, there are still so many skeptics about Prolotherapy. I think it has to be admitted that those in the medical profession, once they have departed from their formal training and have established themselves in practice, are not the most open to innovative and new ideas. Let me give an example. About 15 years after I first met Dr. Hemwall and was treated by him for my lower extremity pain, I began to develop serious pain in my right shoulder girdle and upper arm. I was treated by neck traction, which made me worse, and after sleeping in an awkward position on an airplane to London, I woke up with my right arm paralyzed.

Because of the wonderful care I received at St. Bartholomew's Medical College Hospital, I began to have muscle twitching in my paralyzed arm within three weeks; by six weeks I could open a door and after three months I was back at the operating table. What I learned was that abnormal motion in the skeletal system can produce both sensory and motor symptoms. I had both in my shoulder and arm. I was treated in London by cervical traction, but not as I had been in the United States, just pulling my neck off my shoulders by means of a sling under my chin and my skull, but I was treated by cervical traction with my head flexed forward and turned to one side. That relieved the pressure on the nerves involved and led to my recovery.

When I would have minor symptoms of the same type, I learned from my physiotherapy colleagues in London that the head weighs about 12 pounds and can be used as a means of cervical traction by lying prone on a bed with your shoulders at the edge of a mattress, letting your head hang forward (flexion), and turning it to the side of your pain. There were days that I could barely get my wallet out of my back pocket. I would have to "walk" my fingers across my hip to my pocket and then slowly extricate the wallet. That was my right hand into my right rear pocket. After five minutes of the previously described traction over the edge of a bed, I could put my right arm completely around my back to the other flank.

I was so impressed with what I had learned that, one day, while with a few of my orthopedic and neurosurgical colleagues, I demonstrated the improvement after hanging my head over a gurney outside the operating room. Instead of being impressed, they all walked away as skeptics, some thinking that I had faked the whole thing to impress them.

Prolotherapy is not a cure-all for all pain. Therefore, the diagnosis must be made accurately and the therapy must be done by someone who knows what he or she is doing. The nice thing about Prolotherapy, if properly done, is that it cannot do any harm. How could placing a little sugar-water at the junction of a ligament with a bone be harmful to a patient?

I hope that Dr. Hauser's book, written for laymen, will push them to inquire more about Prolotherapy and that it might receive the place in modern therapeutics that I think it really deserves.

C. Everett Koop, M.D., Sc.D.
Former United States Surgeon General

CHAPTER 1

My Story: What Is a Physiatrist?

I was born on September 14, 1962.... Just joking! You have to learn to relax! Did you know that when we were children we laughed 80 times per day, but as adults we chuckle a measly 15 times per day?! This is especially significant because we do so many funny things.

While attending the University of Illinois Medical School, I had a difficult time deciding on an area of specialization. Family medicine seemed appealing, but working in the intensive care unit was not for me. Then a friend of mine, Steve Primack, now an attending radiologist at the University of Oregon, gave me a book that contained a comprehensive list of medical specialties. After reviewing it and praying with my wife about our future, I decided to look into the field of Physical Medicine and Rehabilitation.

Physical Medicine and Rehabilitation is a medical discipline approved by the American Board of Medical Specialties. After World War II, many soldiers returned home with disabilities, including amputations and spinal cord injuries. Previously, these veterans would have died from infection, but due to the discovery of penicillin they survived their injuries. Unfortunately, physicians had not been trained to care for those suffering from such disabilities. Out of this need eventually came the field of Physical Medicine and Rehabilitation, or Physiatry.

PHYSIATRY

A doctor who specializes in Physical Medicine and Rehabilitation is called a Physiatrist (pronounced *fizz-ee-at-trist*). No, I'm not a Psychiatrist. Look again. Physiatrist. Currently, there are approximately 5,000 board-certified Physiatrists in the United States. Physiatry requires four years of residency training after medical school. Rotations in stroke, multiple sclerosis, traumatic brain injury, amputations, cardiac rehabilitation, electromyography (EMG), spinal cord injury, neurology, sports medicine, orthopedic rehabilitation, and, of course, both acute and chronic pain management are all part of the residency program.

Physiatrists care for patients who suffer from a chronic or acute disease that has affected their ability to enjoy life and perform daily functions. A stroke victim, for example, requires medical attention as well as rehabilitation. Difficulties in blood pressure control, urination, speech, and swallowing are common problems that result from a stroke. Rehabilitation helps the patient relearn how to walk, talk, and live life.

Unfortunately, most people do not consult a Physiatrist because they do not know the profession exists. Even many Family Practice Physicians and Internists are unaware of Physiatry which is probably due to the fact that a rotation in Physical Medicine and Rehabilitation is not mandatory in medical schools. Physiatry is one medical field where a shortage of doctors exists. As man's life-span increases and more people survive disabling diseases, more Physiatrists will be needed.

WHERE IT ALL STARTED

I became fascinated with pain during my Physical Medicine residency. I began accumulating articles on bizarre pain syndromes and obtained quite a collection. (Everyone needs a hobby, right?) What struck me most was the magnitude of the pain problem. It seemed as though everyone either had pain themselves or knew someone who was suffering from chronic pain. I also saw the lack of significant pain relief by modern treatments such as surgery, physical therapy, and anti-inflammatory drugs.

It appeared that the longer people had pain, the less likely such treatments were going to help cure their chronic pain. Pain clinics and pain programs do help some people, but have a poor cure rate. Pain programs teach people to live with their pain. The psychological aspect of the pain is addressed, but in many cases the **cause** is not determined.

When I began seeing pain patients during my residency training program in Physical Medicine and Rehabilitation, I thought they were a very difficult group of people to treat. They often appeared depressed and traditional approaches to pain management did not seem to help. Then I said to myself, "How would I feel if I had pain day after day and no one could find a cure?" The families of many who suffer from pain often begin doubting the reality of their loved one's pain. Many chronic pain patients who frequent pain clinics experience broken homes and lose their jobs because of the pain. It became evident to me that these patients' pain was indeed real and that pain pills and support groups did not cure the pain.

NATURAL MEDICINE

Then came Natural Medicine. I began learning about Natural Medicine the day I married Marion, a dietitian, on December 20, 1986. I watched as my life and surroundings slowly changed. Not long after we moved her things into our condo-minium, (After we were married. We're old fashioned, what can I say?) Marion axed fast-food from my diet. I have not eaten a can of Spaghetti-O's since our wedding. What sacrifices I have made! Marion introduced me to good-tasting spinach and dras-tically altered my diet. The chronic fatigue that I thought was from the intensity of medical training began to subside. I guess the rest is history!

Natural Medicine employs natural substances such as organic foods, herbs, vitamins, and minerals, as well as rest, exercise, and attention to faith in God to maintain and restore health. I began to see that modern medicine was not a cure-all for chronic diseases. Its lack of healing ability was especially evident as it pertained to chronic disabling conditions caused by pain, multiple sclerosis, rheumatoid arthri-tis, and cancer. I knew there had to be something to help all these suffering people.

One of my instructors, Oleh Paly, M.D., gave me a book by Linus Pauling, M.D., on the use of vitamin C in disease. He also directed me to various resources and organizations that specialize in natural healing techniques. This was my first real taste of Natural Medicine.

Soon after, I found myself taking acupuncture lessons and reading up on natural healing techniques. I tried the techniques on my wife. (After I have learned a technique, she always wants to be the first patient.) Since she survived, I tried them out on a few friends. (Most of them are still friends.) A friend from church, Mrs. Wright, was experiencing terrible pain. I tried all the treatment modalities and gizmos I knew of, but without success. Mrs. Wright eventually received treatment from Gustav A. Hemwall, M.D., the world's most experienced Prolotherapist. The Prolotherapy she received in her shoulder gave her a significant amount of relief. Mrs. Wright then encouraged me to learn about Dr. Hemwall's treatment.

PROLOTHERAPY

In April 1992, I contacted Dr. Hemwall and he allowed me to observe him in his clinic. I was astonished to see him perform 30, 40, or 50 injections on a patient at one time! He called his treatment Prolotherapy. The only other time I had come across the term was when a fellow resident showed me a book on the treatment. I later discovered that Dr. Hemwall was one of the authors of that book!

During the next few months, I spent a considerable amount of time in Dr. Hemwall's office. People traveled from all over the world to be treated by this 84-year-old man. I have nothing against age, but to think that someone would travel from places like England, Mexico, Florida, and California to receive pain management was incredible. I learned that if someone suffers from pain and someone else has a technique that will help alleviate the pain, time and expense are minor considerations.

It was clear that Dr. Hemwall was helping those whom traditional medicine had not helped. His average patient had been in pain for years and had tried it all: surgery, pain pills, anti-inflammatory medication, exercise, therapy, acupuncture, and hypnotism. Most patients had seen more than five physicians before consulting Dr. Hemwall. Almost all the patients I observed improved after one or two Prolotherapy treatments. People found relief from pain that had plagued them for years. Many said they wished they had known about Prolotherapy years ago.

Three months later, I began utilizing Prolotherapy in my medical practice as a treatment of chronic pain. I have effectively used Prolotherapy in nearly every joint of the body. In January 1993, I began working alongside Dr. Hemwall in his Prolotherapy practice. Since then, my wife and I have opened Caring Medical and Rehabilitation Services, S.C., a Natural Medicine Clinic that cares for people with chronic diseases using natural methods including Prolotherapy.

Since learning Prolotherapy, the practice of medicine has become more enjoyable. Prolotherapy has enabled me to offer a treatment that eliminates long-standing pain. Chronic pain, like cancer, sucks the lifeblood out of a person. It can disrupt families and lead them into bankruptcy if the pain prohibits the patient from holding a job. What a joy it will be when you or your loved ones find pain relief. I believe this book will lead you, or someone you know, down the path to healing chronic pain naturally with Prolotherapy.

CHAPTER 2

Introduction: The Technique and Its History

N othing was worse than a chronic low back pain patient walking into my office," said Gustav A. Hemwall, M.D., the world's most experienced Prolotherapist. "I would try exercise, corsets, and surgery, but nothing really helped."

In 1955, when Dr. Hemwall visited a scientific exhibit at the national meeting of the American Medical Association, that all changed. Recalling the meeting, Dr. Hemwall said, "At one particular exhibit I noticed a crowd of doctors listening to a doctor say he had a cure for low back pain. This fellow had written a book on it as well." That fellow was George S. Hackett, M.D., the father of Prolotherapy. (*See Appendix E, George S. Hackett AMA Presentations.*)

Once the crowd diminished, Dr. Hemwall asked Dr. Hackett how he could learn the treatment described in his book. Dr. Hackett responded by inviting Dr. Hemwall to observe him administering Prolotherapy. Dr. Hemwall became so proficient at administering the technique that Dr. Hackett would later refer patients to him. **(Figure 2-1)**

Dr. Hemwall remembers, "When I returned from that meeting, I quickly read Dr. Hackett's book describing Prolotherapy and treated my first patient. After a few sessions of Prolotherapy, this patient, instead of coming into the office in a wheelchair, ran to catch four buses. From that point on, instead of dreading patients with low back pain, I began to look for them." That was 40 years ago. Since that time, some 10,000 patients have received Prolotherapy from Dr. Hemwall.

PROLOTHERAPY CASE REPORTS

Chronic low back pain management has taken a drastic turn from when the American Medical Association presented Dr. Hackett's Prolotherapy work at their national meetings in 1955. Now, Prolotherapy is not covered in its journal and is rarely mentioned at national meetings. Unfortunately, for the millions of Americans suffering from chronic back and body pain, several events have led to the reduction in the number of physicians using Prolotherapy.

On August 8, 1959, the *Journal of the American Medical Association* reported a fatality after a Prolotherapy injection series. In the case report, Richard Schneider, M.D., wrote, "...in the instance reported here, it must be emphasized that the sclerosing solution [Prolotherapy solution] was not the usual sodium salt of the vegetable oil fatty acid as described in the original monograph [by Dr. Hackett], but

GEORGE S. HACKETT, M. D.
616 FIRST NATIONAL BANK BUILDING
CANTON 2. OHIO

Jan. 25, 1957

Mrs. Lloyd D. Anderson
315 South 12th Street
Albia, Iowa

Dear Mrs. Anderson:

In reply to your letter of the 21st,
I would suggest that you consult: -

Gustav A. Hemwall, M.D.
839 North Central Avenue
Chicago, Illinois.

Dr. Hemwall is the only man that I
know of in your part of the country who is
experienced with this technic of treatment.
He was out here on several occasions and was
instructed in the technic by me, and I can
recommend him highly.

As to whether your condition could
be benefitted by this procedure, it is
impossible to give you any answer without
first having examined you to determine your
disability.

If I can be of further service,
please feel free to call on me.

Sincerely,

George S. Hackett, M.D.

OSH/mak

Figure 2-1

instead a solution of zinc sulfate in 2.5 percent phenol."[1]

This physician also apparently injected this solution into the spinal canal, not at the fibro-osseous junction where ligaments and tendons attach to bone. Dr. Schneider ended the case report with, "...this technique of precipitating fibro-osseous proliferation appears to be neither sound nor without extreme danger." It should be noted that the article was written by several physicians from the Neurosurgery department at the University of Michigan Hospital.

This tragic case occurred because the physician used too strong a proliferant and did not follow a cardinal rule of Prolotherapy: Prolotherapy injections are given only when the needle is touching the bone at the fibro-osseous junction, with the only exception being joint injections. Unfortunately, early Prolotherapy physicians did not follow Dr. Hackett's technique. The flawed method these physicians utilized caused some harmful effects and discouraged other physicians from administering Prolotherapy. When properly administered, Prolotherapy has no side effects and is effective in eliminating chronic pain.

PROLOTHERAPY SOLUTIONS

In his 19 years of using Sylnasol, a sodium salt of fatty acids and vegetable oil, Dr. Hackett observed no side effects. Dr. Hemwall noted that a number of years after Dr. Hackett's original work was published, Sylnasol was taken off the market due to a lack of demand. After several years of using various solutions, Dr. Hemwall found that a simple Dextrose and Lidocaine solution was the ideal proliferant. It produced only a small amount of pain following the procedure, yet resulted in complete pain relief after only a few treatments. More Dextrose solution could also be injected at one time than with the Sylnasol, allowing more areas of the body to be treated per visit.

It has only been recently that modern medicine has figured out what Dr. Hemwall knew some 35 years ago: that a simple Dextrose solution is all that is needed to eliminate pain. Min-Young Kim, M.D., and associates from Yonsei University Medical College in Seoul, South Korea, studied 64 patients with chronic pain. Dr. Kim compared using a five percent Dextrose solution with the current standard trigger point injection solution of 0.5 percent Lidocaine and placebo. The study found that not only did the Dextrose solution prove to give statistically significant pain relief ($P < .01$) against placebo, it was that much better when compared to the Lidocaine solution. The study also found that in follow-up, the pain relief with the Dextrose solution remained.[2,3]

The Prolotherapy solution I use is 12.5 percent Dextrose, 10.0 percent Sarapin, and 0.2 percent Lidocaine. Dr. Hemwall uses the same solution without the Sarapin. The Dextrose is a corn extract and makes the solution more concentrated than blood (hypertonic), acting as a strong proliferant. Sarapin is used to treat nerve irritation and, in my experience, acts as a proliferant. Sarapin is an extract of the pitcher plant and is one of the few materials listed in the *Physician's Desk Reference* that has no known side effects. Lidocaine is an anesthetic that helps reinforce the diagnosis because the patient will experience immediate pain relief after the Prolotherapy injections.

The current Prolotherapy technique described in this book using these solutions has been administered by Dr. Hemwall and myself to more than 10,000 patients, in more than 40,000 treatment sessions, with more than four million injections given. Not one case of permanent nerve injury, infection, paralysis, or death has been documented. The main side effect has been one to two days of pain after the procedure. The pain is not only from inflammation caused by the Prolotherapy injections, but occurs because the needle pierces the muscle to reach the fibro-osseous junction of the ligaments and tendons being treated.

The Dextrose solution, in addition to being safe, will not affect a diabetic's blood sugar level. If a patient is corn intolerant, other proliferant agents can be used. Such agents include sodium morrhuate (an extract of cod liver oil), preservative-free zinc sulfate, manganese, pumice, or a Dextrose-glycerine-phenol solution known as PG2. Incidentally, PG2 was the proliferant used in the two double-blind studies that will be described in Chapter Four.[4,5]

MYOFASCIAL PAIN THEORY

In the early 1960s, after the damaging report in the *Journal of the American Medical Association*, Janet Travell, M.D., Internist, developed a treatment program for what she termed "Myofascial Pain Syndrome." She noted that patients with chronic pain had tight muscles and after the muscles were stretched or relaxed the pain would diminish. She also described trigger points or areas where muscle is tender to palpation. These trigger points refer pain to other areas of the body. She described these referral pain patterns in detail.[6]

Dr. Travell was an outstanding physician and gave successful care to then Senator John F. Kennedy five years prior to his presidential election. This led to her promotion to White House physician under President Kennedy and President Lyndon B. Johnson. Needless to say, her myofascial pain theory received a great deal of publicity and is embraced today as the main theory for chronic pain management.

Upon examination, the referral pain patterns laid out by Dr. Hackett in 1956 for ligament laxity are strikingly similar to the referral pain patterns described for muscles by Dr. Travell many years later. **(Figure 2-3)** The similarity exists because of the relationship between ligament laxity and muscle tenseness. Ligament weakness causes laxity or looseness in a joint. To stabilize the joint, the muscles tighten up. The overlying muscle is then overworked in an attempt to stabilize the loosened joint. This tense muscle produces trigger points or "knots."

Clinicians who use myofascial stretching techniques for tight muscles often find that the chronic pain is relieved temporarily but returns with the same intensity at some point after treatment. Myofascial therapy often only treats a symptom of the ligament weakness and, because the underlying ligament weakness is not dealt with, pain returns. Prolotherapy, by causing the growth of ligament tissue, treats the root cause of myofascial pain. By strengthening the ligaments, the joint stabilizes, so the muscles have no need to tighten. It is only then that trigger points and muscle tenderness are permanently eliminated.

LOWER BACK AND HIP LIGAMENTS

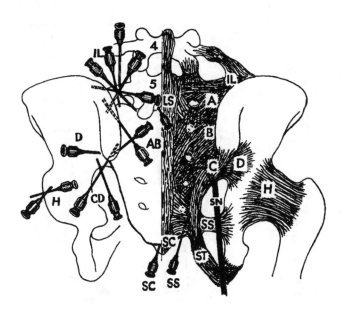

TRIGGER POINTS OF LIGAMENTS

IL -	Iliolumbar
LS -	Lumbosacral - Supra & Interspinus
A, B, C, D -	Posterior Sacroiliac
SS -	Sacrospinus
ST -	Sacrotuberus
SC -	Sacrococcygeal
H -	Hip - Articular
SN -	Sciatic Nerve

Figure 2-2A: Hackett Referral Patterns

Ligamentous structures of the lower back and hip that refer pain down the lower leg. The illustration shows the trigger points of pain and the needles in position for confirmation of the diagnosis and for treatment of ligament relaxation of the lumbosacral and pelvic joints.

PAIN REFERRAL PATTERNS
From Lumbosacral and Pelvic Joint Ligaments

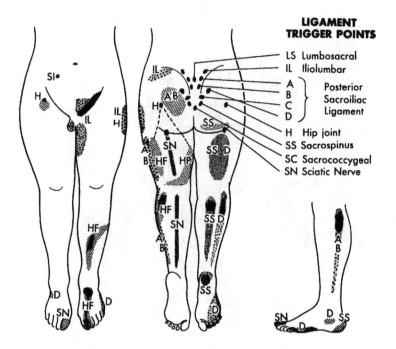

LIGAMENT TRIGGER POINTS

LS Lumbosacral
IL Iliolumbar
A
B } Posterior
C   Sacroiliac
D   Ligament
H   Hip joint
SS Sacrospinus
SC Sacrococcygeal
SN Sciatic Nerve

Referred Pain Areas in the Abdomen, Groin, Genitalia, Buttock, and Extremities from Relaxation of the Posterior Ligaments Which Support the Lumbosacral and Pelvic Joints.

Abbreviation	Ligament	Referral Pattern
IL	Iliolumbar	Groin, Testicles, Vagina, Inner Thigh
AB	Posterior Sacroiliac (upper 2/3rds)	Buttock, Thigh, Leg (outer surface)
D	Posterior Sacroiliac (lower outer fibers)	Thigh, Leg (outer calf), Foot (lateral toes) – Accompanied by Sciatica
HP	Hip – Pelvic Attachment	Thigh – Posterior and Medial
HF	Hip – Femoral Attachment	Thigh – Posterior and Lateral Lower Leg – Anterior And Into the Big Toe and 2nd Toe
SS	Sacrospinus and Sacrotuberus	Thigh – Posterior Lower Leg – Posterior to the Heel
SN	Sciatic Nerve	Can Radiate Pain Down the Leg

Figure 2-2B: Hackett Referral Patterns
Ligament referral pain patterns from structures in Figure 2-2A.

Ligament and Tendon Relaxation Treated by Prolotherapy © 1991, Gustav A. Hemwall, M.D. Used with permission.

HEAD AND NECK REFERRAL PAIN PATTERNS
Ligament and Tendon Relaxation

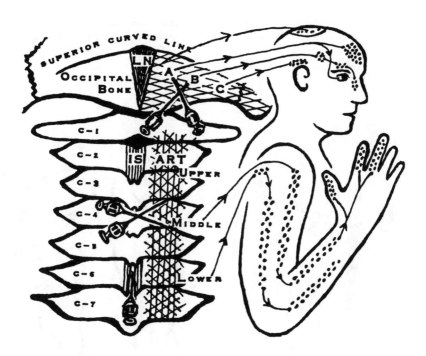

AREA OF WEAKNESS	REFERRAL PATTERN
Occiput Area A	Forehead and Eye
Occiput Area B	Temple, Eyebrow, and Nose
Occiput Area C	Above the Ear
Cervical Vertebrae #1 – #3 (Upper)	Back of Neck and Posterior Scapular Region (Not Shown)
Cervical Vertebrae #4 – #5 (Middle)	Lateral Arm and Forearm Into the Thumb, Index, and Middle Finger
Cervical Vertebrae #6 – #7 (Lower)	Medial Arm and Forearm Into the Lateral Hand, Ring, and Little Finger

Figure 2-2C: Hackett Referral Patterns
Head and neck ligament referral pain patterns.

Ligament and Tendon Relaxation Treated by Prolotherapy © 1991, Gustav A. Hemwall, M.D. Used with permission.

GLUTEUS MEDIUS MUSCLE REFERRAL PATTERN
Janet Travell, M.D.

The gluteus medius muscle refers pain down the lateral leg and into the buttock region.

HIP LIGAMENT REFERRAL PATTERN
George S. Hackett, M.D.

The hip ligaments also refer pain down the lateral leg and into the buttock region.

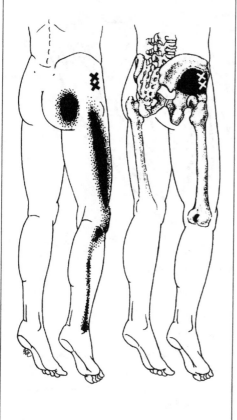

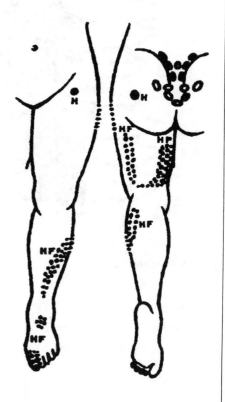

Figure 2-3: Comparison of Travell and Hackett Referral Patterns
Notice the similarities between the referral patterns.

CAT SCANS, MRI SCANS, AND X-RAYS

The next reason for the diminished use of Prolotherapy was the invention of the computerized axial tomography (CAT) scan. The CAT scan became widely available in the early 1970s and was used, among other things, to view the intervertebral disc. Chronic pain physicians in the early 1970s found abnormalities in this area and concluded that the disc problems caused chronic pain. Millions of people underwent surgical procedures to correct some "abnormality" of the disc as seen on the CAT scan, only to experience minimal pain relief.

Not until the early 1980s were the CAT scans of people without pain examined.[7] A study published in 1984 by Sam W. Wiesel, M.D., found that 35 percent of the population, irrespective of age, had abnormal findings on CAT scans of their lower backs even though they had no pain complaints. In CAT scans of people over 40 years of age, 50 percent had abnormal findings. Twenty-nine percent showed evidence of herniated discs, 81 percent facet degeneration (arthritis), and 48 percent lumbar stenosis (another form of arthritis). In other words, for people over 40 years of age who do not have symptoms of pain, a 50 percent chance of abnormality on their CAT scans exists, including a herniated disc.

In regard to pain management, diagnostic tests such as X-rays, magnetic resonance imaging (MRI) scans, or CAT scans should never take the place of a listening ear and a strong thumb to diagnose the cause of chronic pain. It is necessary for the clinician to understand where the pain originates and radiates. In other words, what is the referral pattern? Unfortunately, most physicians do not know the referral patterns of the ligaments, as seen in Figures 2-2. In summary, it should be obvious that an X-ray should not be used solely as the criterion for determining the cause of a person's pain.

To properly diagnose the cause of a person's pain it is important for the physician to touch the patient. Medical doctors are too quick to prescribe an anti-inflammatory medication or order an MRI. The best MRI scan is a physician's thumb, which I call **My** Reproducibility Instrument. I use it to palpate the ligament or tendon suspected to be the problem. If the diagnosis is correct, a positive "jump sign" will occur because the weakened ligament or tendon will be very tender to palpation. If the physician does not reproduce a person's pain during an examination, the likelihood of eliminating the pain is slim. How can a physician make a correct diagnosis without reproducing the pain? Patients often tell me that my initial examination was the first real examination they have had for their pain.

It is not uncommon for a patient to leave my office after the initial consultation, before beginning Prolotherapy treatments, keenly aware of their pain source area. When patients confront me with this, I always smile and say, "What did you expect? You came to a pain doctor!" The point is, a physician must reproduce the pain in order to document the exact pain-producing structure. Once this is located, Prolotherapy injections to strengthen the area will likely eliminate the pain.

THE INSPIRATION FOR THIS BOOK

My inspiration to fulfill my dream of writing this book came in the summer of 1995 when I visited Cornerstone to Health, a Natural Medicine clinic operated by

Gail Gelsinger, R.N. I examined 18 of the clinic's patients who, despite being on a good nutrition program, continued to suffer from chronic pain. I successfully treated each patient with Prolotherapy. When I returned a few months later, twice as many patients desired Prolotherapy treatments. Unfortunately, my schedule prevents me from returning. As a result, a myriad of people needlessly suffer from chronic pain because the treatment of Prolotherapy is unavailable. I then realized how people could benefit from a book about the treatment of chronic pain with Prolotherapy.

Another reason for writing this book is to carry on where Dr. Hemwall has left off. In June 1996, Dr. Hemwall, at the age of 88, retired after 60 years of practicing medicine and 40 years of administering Prolotherapy. Because Dr. Hemwall had the privilege of learning Prolotherapy from its originator, the more books that share his knowledge, the better.

During the 40 years that Dr. Hemwall administered Prolotherapy, he treated more than 10,000 chronic pain patients. One of those 10,000 patients said his pain "originated in my spine, went down across my inguinal ligament, down the inside of my thigh, skipped my knee, went down the inside of my calves, skipped my ankle, and came out the dorsum of my foot like a burn." The patient was describing a sacroiliac referral pattern, and Prolotherapy to the sacroiliac joint very effectively eliminated the pain. This patient would later become the Surgeon General of the United States, C. Everett Koop, M.D.

Dr. Koop says, "I personally know the benefits of Prolotherapy. I had intractable back pain which traveled down my leg. I received Prolotherapy to my back by Dr. Hemwall. After a few treatments, it [the pain] was gone. Seeing the benefits of Prolotherapy on myself, I used the technique on the parents of my patients. I was a pediatric surgeon. When I saw the parents of my patients limping or having trouble taking off their coats, I would offer to treat them with Prolotherapy. I did it all pro bono. Prolotherapy does remarkably well at eliminating the pain caused by ligament relaxation or weakness. For someone experienced in the technique, it is extremely safe and effective. I utilized the technique of Prolotherapy from 1960 to 1980 and found it extremely effective in eliminating the chronic pain that comes from ligament relaxation."[8]

For the past 25 years, Dr. Hemwall has been the main proponent and teacher of Prolotherapy in the United States. He is responsible for training more physicians and treating more people with Prolotherapy than anyone else. Without his perseverance, the Hackett technique of Prolotherapy may have vanished. During the past five years, I have been blessed to have worked under him as a student, with him as a partner, and beside him as a colleague. In this book, I hope to disseminate what I have gleaned from a man I very much admire.

THE WEAKNESS OF MODERN MEDICINE

While a wonderful and effective procedure known as Prolotherapy has been achieving pain relief for more than 50 years, modern medicine continues to search for drugs, devices, and surgical procedures to eliminate chronic pain. Anti-inflammatory drugs have become a multibillion dollar business. While these drugs provide temporary relief, they do not correct the underlying condition causing the pain. Migraine headaches are not caused by an ibuprofen deficiency. When these drugs do not give permanent relief, the next step is typically exercise or physical therapy. As with the drugs, physical therapy and exercise provide temporary relief for the pain during the therapy, but the pain often returns once the therapy concludes.

The next step down the wrong path for the chronic pain patient is a referral to a surgeon. Unfortunately for many, surgery has not been the promised end to their pain and often makes the problem worse. Surgeons often use X-ray technology as a diagnostic tool. This is often not appropriate to properly diagnose the pain source. It is not uncommon for an X-ray to reveal terrible arthritis in someone who experiences no symptoms, whereas an X-ray of someone who has terrible pain symptoms may reveal nothing.

After examining these X-rays, a surgeon may decide to remove a disc or cartilage tissue in an attempt to alleviate pain. The two questions to ask are: Who put that tissue there? For what purpose? I believe God placed disc tissue there to stabilize and cushion the lower back, and cartilage tissue in the joints so that bones glide smoothly over one another. What happens when the disc and cartilage tissue are removed? If the disc is removed, the vertebral levels above and below the surgerized segment develop proliferative arthritis. This is due to these segments having to carry more of the force than they were designed to carry in the lower back. If the cartilage is removed, the bones no longer glide smoothly over one another. Soon after this, a person notices a crunching of the joint where the cartilage was removed. This crunching sound is arthritis. The end result of surgical procedures that remove cartilage, ligaments, and bone from knees, backs, and necks is often arthritis.

Unfortunately, medicine has lost the art of clinical diagnosis without the aid of fancy tests and machines. Prolotherapists (physicians who practice Prolotherapy) are trained to reproduce and effectively treat a painful area without the need for X-rays or expensive tests.

PROLOTHERAPY AS PAIN MANAGEMENT

Other unnatural, ineffective, and/or destructive means to relieve pain include the implantation of a spinal cord stimulator, botulism toxin injections into muscles, and radiofrequency thermocoagulation of nerves and other bodily structures. These treatments sound impressive but end up changing or destroying God-given anatomy or other bodily processes often without a long-term cure of the painful condition. Chronic pain is not due to a spinal cord stimulator or botulism toxin deficiency. A more sensible, natural approach to pain management would be to repair the damaged weakened tissue. Chronic pain is almost always due to a weakened damaged tissue. A herniated disc, for example, is better treated by allowing the regrowth of ligament tissue through which the disc herniated, than by removing the disc.

Nathaniel W. Boyd's book, *Stay Out of the Hospital*, describes ligament relaxation. "Once forcibly stretched by trauma, ligamentous tissue is unable to snap back to its original length. This being the case, it should not be very difficult to understand how the ligaments of any joint, once overstretched, will leave the joint wobbly, loose, and in an unstable condition. Along with this instability very often comes chronic pain. The object of 'needle surgery' in treating unstable joints is to inject a sclerosing agent into the ligaments, causing the contraction and thickening of the ligament, thus strengthening its supporting effect on that joint." Boyd is describing Prolotherapy.[9]

Boyd continues by saying that the cause of back pain in a so-called ruptured disc is not pressure of the disc on nerve roots, as orthopedic surgeons would have you believe, because the disc is absorbed by the body in a few weeks. The back hurts in such cases, because once the disc has disappeared, the spinal column loses vertical height and the ligaments become too long and loose to keep the structure stable. This instability and unwanted motion create core irritation, congestion, and inflammation.[10]

Surgery and other invasive treatments are directed at relieving pain but not relieving the underlying condition that caused the pain in the first place. What happens when you cover up a problem and do not solve it? Can you imagine "solving" your financial problems by paying your bills with your credit card? By doing so, your financial problems actually worsen. When treatments cover up the pain without correcting the underlying problem, the initial condition that caused the pain may actually worsen. The person may require more and more pain medicine or other treatments in order to alleviate the pain. I hope that by educating more patients and physicians about Prolotherapy we can end the onslaught of these procedures and correct the "true" underlying cause of the pain.

CHAPTER 3

Why Prolotherapy Works

"A joint is only as strong as its weakest ligament." — George S. Hackett, M.D.

S imply put, **pain is due to weakness**. If my buddy Joe and I were to pick up a piano, I can guarantee we wouldn't be holding it long. After a few seconds, Joe's back would be hurting and about everything on me would be aching. We would be in pain because, unlike Hercules, we are too weak to lift a piano. Likewise, most neck, back, and other musculoskeletal pains are due to weakness, specifically weakness in the ligaments and tendons.

"Ligament relaxation is a condition in which the strength of the ligament fibers has become impaired so that a stretching of the fibrous strands occurs when the ligament is submitted to normal or less than normal tension."[1] This statement was made 40 years ago by George S. Hackett, M.D., who believed chronic pain was simply due to ligament weakness in and around the joint. Dr. Hackett coined the phrase "ligament and tendon relaxation" which is synonymous with ligament and tendon weakness, and subsequently developed the treatment known as Prolotherapy.

PROLOTHERAPY DEFINED

Webster's Third New International Dictionary defines Prolotherapy as "the rehabilitation of an incompetent structure, such as a ligament or tendon, by the induced proliferation of new cells."[2] Prolotherapy is the injection of substances at the site where ligaments and tendons attach to the bone, thus stimulating the ligaments and tendons to proliferate or grow at the injection site. This area is called the fibro-osseous junction. "Fibro" means fibrous tissue which forms the ligament or tendon, and "osseous" refers to the bone.

Prolotherapy works because it addresses and corrects the root cause of chronic pain: ligament and tendon relaxation.

LIGAMENTS AND TENDONS

A **strain** is defined as a stretched or injured tendon. A **sprain** is a stretched or injured ligament. Blood flow is vital to the body's healing process and, because ligaments and tendons have naturally poor blood supply, incomplete healing may result after an injury to that structure.[3,4] This incomplete healing results in decreased strength of the area. The ligaments and tendons, normally taut and thus strong bands of fibrous or connective tissue, become relaxed and weak. The weakened ligament or tendon then becomes the source of the chronic pain.

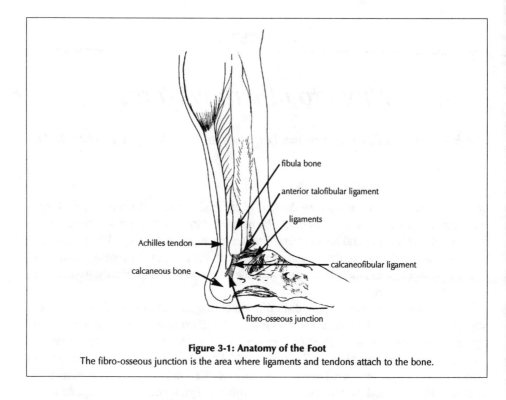

Figure 3-1: Anatomy of the Foot
The fibro-osseous junction is the area where ligaments and tendons attach to the bone.

Ligaments and tendons are bands of tissue consisting of various amino acids in a matrix called collagen. Tendons attach the muscles to the surface of the bone, enabling movement of the joints and bones. Ligaments attach one bone to another, thus preventing overextension of bones and joints. **(Figure 3-1)**

Damage to ligaments and tendons will cause excessive movement of the joints resulting in chronic pain. Damage to ligaments causes joints to become loose or weak and often manifests itself with a cracking sensation during movement. Tendon weakness produces painful and weak joints.

For example, there are many causes of chronic elbow pain including the tennis elbow (extensor tendonitis), annular ligament sprain, and biceps muscle strain. Since muscle, ligament, or tendon injury can all cause pain, a proper diagnosis is needed to permanently alleviate the pain. Tennis elbow is diagnosed when the physician notices weakness and pain with wrist extension and tenderness at the elbow where the extensor tendons attach. Annular ligament sprain is diagnosed by the physician palpating this ligament in the elbow and eliciting a positive "jump sign." **(Figure 3-2)**

Another source of elbow pain is biceps muscle strain. When the biceps tendon is weak, resisted flexion (resisting the upward movement of the forearm) of the elbow is painful. Since the bicep muscle flexes at the elbow, carrying a box or turning a screwdriver may produce the painful symptoms associated with strain or weakness of this muscle. Since the extensor tendons, bicep muscle, and annular ligament

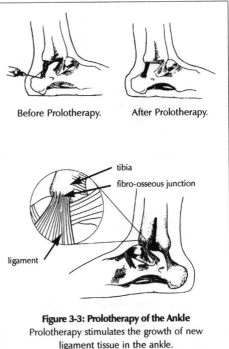

Before Prolotherapy.   After Prolotherapy.

tibia
fibro-osseous junction

ligament

Figure 3-3: Prolotherapy of the Ankle
Prolotherapy stimulates the growth of new
ligament tissue in the ankle.

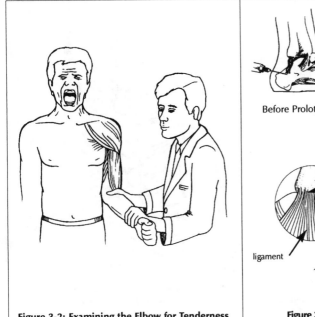

Figure 3-2: Examining the Elbow for Tenderness
Physician elicits a positive "jump sign" while
palpating the annular ligament.

all attach to the bone in the elbow, good palpatory skills are necessary for proper diagnosis. Prolotherapy is given at the fibro-osseous junction where the positive "jump sign" is elicited. Prolotherapy causes proliferation, or growth, of tissue at this point. **(Figure 3-3)** Prolotherapy will strengthen the muscle, tendon, or ligament tissue at the fibro-osseous junction which is needed to alleviate pain.

WHAT ARE LIGAMENTS AND TENDONS?

The most sensitive structures that produce pain according to Daniel Kayfetz, M.D., are the periosteum and the ligaments. It is important to note that in the scale of pain sensitivity (which part of the body hurts more when injured), Dr. Kayfetz notes that the periosteum (outer layer of bone) ranks first, followed by ligaments, tendons, fascia (the connective tissue that surrounds muscle), and finally muscle. Articular (joint) cartilage contains no sensory nerve endings. The area where the ligaments attach to the bone is the fibro-osseous junction. This is why injury to this area is so significant. It causes massive amounts of pain. This is where the Prolotherapy injections occur and thus the strengthening of these areas and subsequent relief of pain.[5]

Ligaments provide stability of the joints. If joints move too much, the bones may compress or pinch nerves or blood vessels resulting in permanent nerve damage. Weakened structures are strengthened by the growth of **new**, strong ligament and tendon tissue induced by the Prolotherapy injections. This is illustrated in a relatively

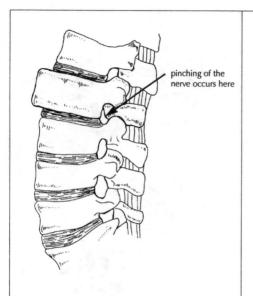

**Figure 3-4A: Spondylolisthesis - Slippage
of the Vertebrae**
Weakened ligaments lead to
spondylolisthesis and pinching of the nerves.

pinching of the
nerve occurs here

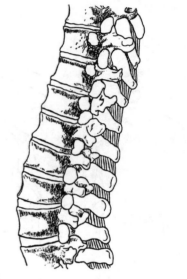

**Figure 3-4B: Proper Vertebral Alignment
After Prolotherapy**
Prolotherapy strengthens the ligaments and joints that
support the vertebrae causing the vertebrae to move
into proper alignment and relieves nerve pinching.

common back condition called spondylolisthesis. A weak area of bone, in conjunction with stretched ligaments, allow vertebrae to slip and pinch a nerve, resulting in terrible back pain and radiating pain down the leg. Prolotherapy strengthens the weakened areas and realigns the vertebrae, relieving the pinched nerve and eliminating the chronic pain. **(Figures 3-4)**

THE ROLE OF PROLOTHERAPY

Prolotherapy permanently strengthens tissue. Strengthening weakened structures produces permanent pain relief. Prolotherapy effectively eliminates pain because it attacks the source of the pain: the fibro-osseous junction, an area rich in sensory nerves.[6,7] When a weakened ligament or tendon is stretched, the sensory nerves become irritated, causing local and referred pain throughout the body. These referred pain patterns of ligaments were outlined in Dr. Hackett's observations after he performed more than 18,000 intraligamentous injections to 1,656 patients over a period of 19 years.[8]

A referred pain occurs when a local ligament injury sends pain to another area of the body. Dr. Hackett described the referral patterns of the ligaments involving the hip, pelvis, lower back, and neck. (*See Figures 2-2.*) Physical therapists, chiropractors, family physicians, and orthopedists are usually unaware of ligament referral pain patterns. From the illustration, note that the hip ligaments refer pain to the big toe. The sacroiliac ligaments refer pain to the lateral foot, which causes the symptoms resulting in a common misdiagnosis of "sciatica." Pain traveling down the back into the leg and foot is usually from ligament weakness in the sacroiliac joint, not pinching of the sciatic nerve. Patients who are misdiagnosed with "sciatica" are often subjected to numerous tests, anti-inflammatory medicines, and surgical procedures with unsatisfactory results. Prolotherapy eliminates the local ligament pain, as well as the referred pain, and is curative in most cases of sciatica.

Ligament injuries may cause crushing severe pain because the ligaments are full of nerves, some of the nerve tissue being free nerve endings.[9,10] Movement may aggravate the damaged nerve in the ligament and produces a shock-like sensation, giving the impression that a nerve is being pinched. It is a nerve-type pain that is due to a ligament stretching, not a nerve pinching. When a weak ligament is stretched, the nerves inside the ligament often send shock-like pain to distant sites, as in sciatica pain. If the ligament is strengthened with Prolotherapy, the nerves in the ligaments do not fire, thereby relieving the pain.

It is well-known that an injury in one segment of the body can affect other distant body parts, especially in regard to ligament injury. For example, when dye is injected into the nerves of the ligaments of the lower neck, the dye will travel four segments above and four segments below the initial injection site. The dye may be seen in the autonomic (sympathetic) nerves in these areas.[11] This implies that ligament laxity at one vertebral level could manifest pain, muscle tension, adrenal, or automatic dysfunction four segments above or below the actual injury site. This is one of the explanations as to why ligament pain is often diffuse and can take on a burning quality.

Knowledge of referral pain patterns, along with a complete patient medical history, allows physicians who practice Prolotherapy to make accurate diagnoses of specific weak ligaments, even before performing an examination. A Prolotherapist, for example, may examine a back pain patient with pain radiating down the leg to the knee. This reveals that the source of the pain is likely the "A" and "B" areas of the sacroiliac ligaments. (*As seen in Figures 2-2A and 2-2B.*) Pain continuing to the lateral foot indicates weak "D" area sacroiliac ligaments. Pain radiating to the big toe reveals the source is in the hip area.

The physician examines the appropriate area utilizing his most important diagnostic tool—the thumb. I call it my personal MRI scanner: **M**y **R**eproducibility **I**nstrument. A diagnosis is made when a positive "jump sign" is observed. This occurs when the injured ligament is palpated, causing the patient to jump off the examination table due to the severe tenderness of the ligament. The pain is caused by something between the pressing thumb and the bone. The something between these two areas is the ligament. **(Figure 3-5)** The positive "jump sign" gives both patient and physician confidence that the pain-producing structure has been identified. Ligament injuries are often not detected with CAT or MRI scans because ligaments are such small structures. If a positive "jump sign" can be elicited, then permanent pain relief with Prolotherapy is likely.

Prolotherapy is so successful because it attacks the root cause of chronic pain which is most commonly ligament laxity (weakness). Signs of ligament laxity or

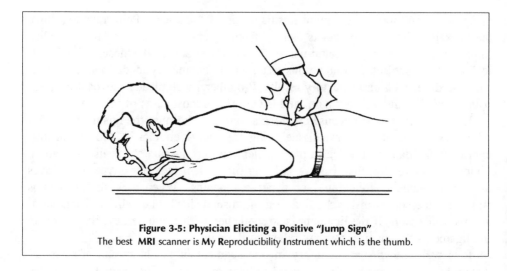

Figure 3-5: Physician Eliciting a Positive "Jump Sign"
The best MRI scanner is My Reproducibility Instrument which is the thumb.

injury are the following: 1) chronic pain, 2) referral pain patterns, 3) tender areas, 4) positive "jump signs," 5) pain aggravated by movement, 6) cracking sensation in the joint when moved, 7) chronic subluxation, or 8) temporary help from physical therapy, massage, or chiropractic manipulation. Prolotherapy helps strengthen chronically weak ligaments and relieves all of the above.

In summary, Prolotherapy works by permanently strengthening the ligament, muscle, and tendon attachments to the bone, the fibro-osseous junction. Because the cause of pain is addressed, Prolotherapy is often curative.

CHAPTER 4

Prolotherapy Provides Results

Prolotherapy is effective because it attacks and eliminates the root cause of chronic pain: ligament and tendon relaxation. Ligament relaxation causes joints to loosen. A weak ligament will have difficulty holding a joint in place. The nerve fibers within the weakened ligament are activated and cause local pain. They may also cause a referred pain pattern as shown in Figures 2-2. The muscles surrounding the loose ligament contract to help stabilize the joint—the reason why people with loose ligaments and chronic pain have tight, painful muscles. Only when the weakened ligaments are strengthened will the local and referred pain patterns, as well as the muscle pain, subside. The same is true for tendon weakness.

Research has been conducted exhibiting the effectiveness of Prolotherapy. The following studies are just a sample of the research that has been done during the past 40 years.

GEORGE S. HACKETT, M.D.

Although chronic pain has many causes, the vast majority of chronic pain sufferers have loose joints caused by ligament weakness. This is evidenced by George S. Hackett, M.D.'s research study described in the third edition of his book, *Ligament and Tendon Relaxation Treated by Prolotherapy*, published in 1958.[1] The study consisted of the following:

- sample size: 656 patients
- patient age range: 15 to 88 years old
- duration of pain prior to treatment: three months to 65 years
- average duration of pain prior to treatment: four-and-a-half years
- duration of study: 19 years
- number of injections given: 18,000

Twelve years after the Prolotherapy treatment was completed, 82 percent of the patients considered themselves cured. Dr. Hackett believed that the cure rate with Prolotherapy was over 90 percent due to improvements in the technique over the years.

In 1955, Dr. Hackett analyzed 146 consecutive cases of undiagnosed low back disability during a two-month period. He found that 94 percent of the patients experienced joint ligament relaxation. In 1956, a similar survey of 124 consecutive cases of undiagnosed low back disability revealed that 97 percent of patients possessed joint instability from ligament weakness. The sacroiliac ligaments were involved in 75 percent of the low back ligament laxity cases. The lumbosacral ligaments were involved in 54 percent. He also noted that approximately 50 percent had already undergone back surgery for a previous diagnosis of a disc problem.[2]

At this time, Prolotherapy produced an 80 percent cure rate even though 50 percent of the people treated had undergone back surgery. Obviously, the surgical procedures did not relieve the patients' back pain. Rarely does a disc problem cause disabling back pain. (*See Chapter Seven, Prolo Your Back Pain Away.*) Chronic pain in the lower back is most commonly due to ligament weakness—the reason Prolotherapy is so effective.

Dr. Hackett attributed ineffective response to Prolotherapy to: 1) inability to clearly confirm the diagnosis by the injection of a local anesthetic solution, 2) failure of the patient to return for completion of the treatment, 3) treatment in the presence of another disability, 4) a less refined technique and less experience in the earlier studies, 5) lowered morale from years of suffering and disappointment from unsuccessful treatments and dependence on prescription pain medications, and 6) nonresponsiveness to the stimulation of proliferation.

Prolotherapy works because it causes ligament and tendon growth. Dr. Hackett used Sylnasol, a sodium salt fatty acid, as a proliferant in his original work. Animals were given between one and three injections of the proliferating solution into the tendon and the fibro-osseous junction. There was no necrosis (dead tissue) noted in any of the specimens. No destruction of nerves, blood vessels, or tendinous bands was noted. Compared to noninjected tendons, tendons treated with Prolotherapy showed a 40 percent increase in diameter. The fibro-osseous junction, where the tendon attaches to bone, increased by 30 percent, forming permanent tendon tissue. Dr. Hackett believed the 40 percent increase in diameter of the tendon represented a doubling of the tendon strength.[3]

GUSTAV A. HEMWALL, M.D.

Gustav A. Hemwall, M.D., learned the technique of Prolotherapy from Dr. Hackett and then proceeded to treat more than 10,000 patients worldwide. He collected data on 8,000 of those patients. In 1974, Dr. Hemwall presented his largest survey of 2,007 Prolotherapy patients to the Prolotherapy Association. The survey related the following:
- 1,871 patients completed treatment
- 6,000 Prolotherapy treatments were administered
- 1,399 (75.5 percent) patients reported complete recovery and cure
- 413 (24.3 percent) reported general improvement
- 25 (0.2 percent) patients showed no improvement
- 170 patients were lost to follow-up

More than 99 percent of the patients who completed treatment with Prolotherapy found relief from their chronic pain. These results are similar to those published by Dr. Hackett, showing that Prolotherapy is completely curative in many cases and provides some pain relief in nearly all.[4]

Y. KING LIU, PH.D.

In 1983, Y. King Liu performed a study using the knee ligament in rabbits.[5] This study was done to confirm Dr. Hackett's earlier work and better quantify the strength of the tissue formed by Prolotherapy. In this study, a five percent sodium morrhuate solution, an extract of cod liver oil, was injected into the femoral and tibial attachments of the medial collateral ligament, the inside knee ligament.

The ligaments were injected five times and then compared to noninjected ligaments. The results showed that in every case **Prolotherapy significantly increased** ligamentous mass, thickness, and cross-sectional area as well as the ligament strength. In a six-week period, ligament mass increased by 44 percent, ligament thickness by 27 percent, and the ligament-bone junction strength by 28 percent. This research was yet another attestation to the effectiveness of Prolotherapy, showing that Prolotherapy actually causes new tissue to grow.

J. A. MAYNARD, M.D.

To confirm the work of Dr. Liu and describe how the proliferants in Prolotherapy grow tissue, J.A. Maynard, M.D., and associates, treated rabbit tendons with proliferant solutions. After the proliferant injections, the actual tendon circumferences increased an average of 20 to 25 percent after six weeks.

They found that "the increase in circumference appeared to be due to an increase in cell population [immune cells], water content, and ground substance [glue that holds the collagen together].... Consequently, not only is there an increase in the number of cells but also a wider variety of cell types, fibroblasts, neutrophils, lymphocytes, plasma cells, and unidentifiable cells in the injected tissues."[6]

The findings were similar to what normally occurs when injured tissue is repairing itself. Prolotherapy induces the **normal** healing mechanisms of the body. After Prolotherapy, there is increased circulation bringing with it not only nutrients, but cells. These immune cells then begin the growth of collagen tissue to rebuild the injured tissue. Eventually, new collagen tissue forms, creating stronger ligaments and tendons.[7]

ROBERT KLEIN, M.D.

In human studies, Robert Klein, M.D., and associates, administered a series of six weekly injections in the lower back ligamentous supporting structures with a proliferant solution containing Dextrose, glycerin, and phenol. Biopsies performed three months after completion of injections showed statistically significant increases in collagen fiber and ligament diameter by 60 percent. Statistically significant improvements in pain relief and back motion were also observed.[8]

THOMAS DORMAN, M.D.

In a 1989 study, Thomas Dorman, M.D., noted, "I biopsied individuals before and after treatment with Prolotherapy and submitted the biopsy specimens to pathologists. Using modern analytic techniques, they showed that Prolotherapy caused regrowth of tissue, an increased number of fibroblast nuclei, (the major cell type in ligaments and other connective tissue), an increased amount of collagen, and an absence of inflammatory changes or other types of tissue damage."[9]

Dr. Dorman performed a retrospective survey of 80 patients treated with Prolotherapy for cervical, thoracic, lumbar spine pain, or a combination of these. Thirty-one percent of the patients had litigation or workman's compensation cases. The patients were evaluated up to five years after their Prolotherapy treatment. Analysis of the 80 patients showed a statistical significance of $P < .001$ for improvements in 1) severity of pain, 2) daily living activities, and 3) influence of sleep pattern. Prolotherapy was shown to eliminate pain, improve activity level, and help the patients get a good night's sleep.[10]

MILNE ONGLEY, M.D.

Using the same solution as Dr. Klein, Milne Ongley, M.D., and associates, demonstrated a stabilization of the collateral and cruciate ligaments of the knee joint with Prolotherapy. All subjects treated showed an increase in activity and reduction in pain.[11] Two double-blind studies where patients received either a proliferant injected solution or a solution without proliferant concluded that Prolotherapy was effective in eliminating pain.[12,13]

A problem with controlled studies using Prolotherapy injections is that the control group still receives an injection, though without any proliferant. An injection into a tender area is a treatment utilized in pain management. The result is that the control group actually receives a therapeutic intervention. Despite these concerns, Prolotherapy in the above two studies was shown to be an effective treatment for chronic low back pain.

ROBERT SCHWARTZ, M.D.

In another study, by Robert Schwartz, M.D., on the effects of Prolotherapy on 43 patients with chronic low back pain who had been unresponsive to other treatments including surgery, Prolotherapy treatments were given over a six-week period into and around the sacroiliac joint. At two weeks, 20 of 43 patients reported 95 percent improvement, 31 of 43 patients reported 75 percent or better improvement, and 35 of 43 reported 66 percent or better improvement. Only three of 43 reported no improvement. The result of this study of chronic resistant low back pain, revealed that 93 percent of the patients experienced pain relief with Prolotherapy after the six weeks.[14]

HAROLD WILKINSON, M.D.

Between 1979 and 1995, Harold Wilkinson, M.D., a professor and former chairman of the Division of Neurosurgery at the University of Massachusetts Medical Center who has been practicing Prolotherapy for 30 years, gave 349 posterior iliac Prolotherapy injections for chronic low back pain. Generally, the patients had undergone prior spinal operations and had been referred to him because they were "failed back patients." In other words, no one could help them. Of the 349 injections, one injection totally relieved 29 percent of the patients, and a total of 76 percent of the patients received significant pain relief with one injection. A full 93 percent of the people received pain relief with only **one** Prolotherapy injection in the lower back.[15]

In regard to other areas of the body besides the lower back, Dr. Wilkinson reported on results of 115 Prolotherapy injections. Forty-three percent of these completely eliminated the person's pain and 89 percent of the patients, with only one Prolotherapy injection, received some pain relief. Dr. Wilkinson, in compiling the data, stated that it was noteworthy that "a sizeable portion of people with unresolved chronic pain had more than a year's pain relief with only one Prolotherapy injection."

Dr. Wilkinson explained that exercise and massage help trigger points (tender points) originating from muscles by increasing blood circulation but these treatments do not help ligamentous or periosteal (fibro-osseous) trigger points. This is because just increasing blood circulation is not enough to grow the new ligament tissue. Prolotherapy must be done to stimulate the growth of ligamentous tissue at the periosteal junction.

CONFIRMING DIAGNOSIS

There are two aspects by which the correct diagnosis can be completely and reliably confirmed without extensive tests. The first method involves palpating the area involved until a positive "jump sign" is elicited. If a patient's pain can be reproduced by manual palpation, the prognosis for complete relief with Prolotherapy is excellent.

The second method of confirming the diagnosis is by the Prolotherapy treatment itself. The Prolotherapy solution contains various proliferants along with an anesthetic. Prolotherapy is one of the few treatments that actually treats the condition while confirming the diagnosis. Since Prolotherapy injections are given where the ligaments and tendons attach to the bone (fibro-osseous junction) the patient will feel immediate pain relief after the treatment, if the diagnosis is correct. This is due to the effect of the local anesthetic blocking the pain coming from the injured ligaments and tendons. Immediate pain relief after Prolotherapy treatments, along with the reproducibility of the pain when the ligament or tendon is palpated, gives both the patient and the physician confidence that the diagnosis of ligament and tendon relaxation is correct.

SUMMARY

Prolotherapy works because an accurate diagnosis of ligament and tendon weakness can be confirmed by an appropriate patient history and a reproduction of the pain by direct palpation of the injured structure. The pain is immediately alleviated due to the effect of the anesthetic from the Prolotherapy solution. This provides further confirmation that the diagnosis of ligament and tendon relaxation is correct.

Prolotherapy causes a thickening of ligament and tendon tissue. This increases the strength of the ligament and tendon and causes the chronic pain to subside. According to Dr. Hackett and Dr. Hemwall, Prolotherapy is more than 90 percent effective in either eliminating chronic pain or significantly decreasing pain complaints. It is for these reasons that many people are choosing to Prolo their chronic pain away.

CHAPTER 5

Answers to Common Questions About Prolotherapy

A fter years of suffering from chronic pain, many people find it hard to believe that there is a treatment they haven't heard about, that it has the potential to cure them, and on top of it, has been around for 50 years. As hard as it is to believe, there is a treatment that can cure chronic pain and yes, Prolotherapy has been around for 50 years.

I enjoy questions. I once asked my wife if she thought I was the greatest. She replied, "You're the greatest person I know to get us into a fiasco." That was not the answer I was looking for! Anyone contemplating any procedure, including Prolotherapy, should have all of their questions answered. They should also understand why they are getting the procedure and what it is supposed to accomplish.

1. DO PROLOTHERAPY INJECTIONS HURT?

As the saying goes with body builders, it also goes with Prolotherapy, "no pain, no gain." Shots are shots. "Do they hurt?" every new patient asks, as sweat begins to form on the patient's forehead and palms as the needle approaches its target. Let me put it to you this way, my patients begin to sweat when they see me in the grocery store. I don't know why, I'm a nice guy! I think all doctors were taught the appropriate answer to this question in medical school. "It hurts a little." Does anything the doctor sticks you with really hurt just a little? Some people have many Prolotherapy injections and do not flinch, while others receive a few shots and have a rough time.

A good friend and an expert in Orthopedic Medicine, Rodney Van Pelt, M.D., told me the following story about his first Prolotherapy experience. He once attended a conference where Gustav A. Hemwall, M.D., the world's most experienced Prolotherapist, discussed the technique and asked for a volunteer to help illustrate an actual Prolotherapy procedure. So, Dr. Van Pelt, being the adventuresome Californian that he is, jumped out of his seat and volunteered.

For many years, Dr. Van Pelt had suffered from back pain without finding a curative treatment. Due to the deteriorated state of his back, he required quite a number of Prolotherapy injections. Before Dr. Hemwall had finished the treatment, the pain from the injections caused Dr. Van Pelt to pass out. Dr. Hemwall just went on injecting and instructing the physicians on the use of Prolotherapy for chronic low back pain. He then informed the audience that he would rather treat 100 women than one man.

Let's face it. God made women to be able to deliver babies. It has been said that if men were to deliver babies, the human race would become extinct. The amount of pain experienced during the Prolotherapy treatment is insignificant compared to the pain the chronic pain patient experiences every day. Many say after the Prolotherapy treatment, "It wasn't that bad." There are a few people, however, like Dr. Van Pelt, who need a little pampering.

Pampering to lessen the pain may consist of the physician giving the patient anesthesia or a prescription for Tylenol with codeine or Vicodin to be taken prior to Prolotherapy treatments. Other physicians, including Dr. Hemwall and myself, use a device called Madajet which sprays an anesthetic such as Lidocaine into the skin to deaden the pain when the needle pierces the skin. The needle piercing through the skin is the most painful part of the procedure.

For those requiring injections in many areas at one time or in very delicate areas like the neck, intravenous anesthesia such as Demerol, a narcotic, is used. The intravenous anesthesia is the most dangerous part of the procedure. An occasional nausea and a few "upchucks" were the only side effects Dr. Hemwall witnessed after administering thousands of intravenous anesthetics. The anesthesia does make a person "woozy" but most people prefer it because it eliminates the pain of the procedure.

2. HOW SAFE IS PROLOTHERAPY?

In his study published in 1961, Abraham Myers, M.D., states that in treating 267 patients with low back pain with and without sciatica from May 1956 to October 1960 "over 4,500 [Prolotherapy] injections have been given without the occurrence of any complication."[1]

Prolotherapy is much safer than taking aspirin day after day. Prolotherapy is also much safer for the body than living with pain. The most dangerous part of receiving Prolotherapy treatments at my office is fighting Chicago traffic!

Pain not only decreases one's enjoyment of life, it creates stress in the body. Stress is the worst detriment to good health. A body under stress triggers the "fight or flight" response, which means the adrenal gland begins excreting hormones, such as cortisol and adrenaline. The same thing occurs when a gun is pointed at you during a robbery, but for a shorter period of time.

The adrenal gland, also known as the stress gland, secretes cortisol to increase the amount of white blood cells that are activated, as in cases of allergic or infectious stress. It puts the body "on alert." The adrenal gland is one of the reasons a person wakes up in the morning. Chronic pain causes the adrenal gland to be in a continual "alert mode," secreting cortisol as would occur with an infection, or when a person is being robbed. As the chronic pain lingers, cortisol is continually produced. Cortisol levels are supposed to be low at night time, putting the body in the sleep mode. With chronic pain, high cortisol levels put the body in the alert mode and insomnia results. The increased cortisol production eventually wears the body down, resulting in increased fatigue. This explains why many chronic pain patients have difficulty sleeping and complain of nonrestful sleep.

The adrenal gland also secretes adrenaline, more properly named epinephrine, which is the hormone that stimulates the sympathetic nervous system. When the sympathetic nervous system is activated, blood vessels constrict and blood pressure rises—an unhealthy situation long-term. This produces free radicals, causing oxidative damage to the body. Long-term stress from chronic pain results in long-term oxidative damage. This is one reason that people who suffer from chronic pain are ill more frequently and age prematurely. This can also explain why they seem "stressed out." Physiologically, they are! For chronic pain patients, the only way to turn off the adrenaline system is to eliminate the pain. If the chronic pain is due to ligament or tendon laxity, Prolotherapy is required.

Pain causes enormous stress on the body which further enhances the need to rid the body of the pain. Prolotherapy is recommended for every patient with structural chronic pain. Structural pain from a loose joint, cartilage, muscle, tendon, or ligament weakness can be eliminated with Prolotherapy.

Dr. Hemwall, who has treated more than 10,000 patients with more than four million injections, has not had one episode of paralysis, death, permanent nerve injury, or infection. In the words of Dr. Hemwall, "not even a pimple" has formed at the site of the injections. It is common, however, to experience muscle stiffness after the injections for a few days.

3. WHAT ABOUT PRESCRIPTION NARCOTICS?

Dr. Hemwall prescribes analgesics like Tylenol with codeine to ease stiffness and pain after Prolotherapy treatments. I occasionally use codeine, but I more commonly use Tylenol, Ultram (which do not decrease inflammation), or natural analgesics like bromelain or natural muscle relaxers such as magnesium. I do not recommend chronic use of narcotic medications like codeine, Vicodin, or Darvocet. These are wonderful pain killers, but chronic pain is never due to a Tylenol with codeine deficiency. Chronic pain always has a cause. If that cause is eliminated, the pain will disappear.

Most people understand the addictive quality of narcotics. This is a good reason not to use narcotics for more than a few days. Another reason to avoid narcotics is that narcotic medications suppress the immune system.

Chronic use of narcotics has been shown to decrease both B-cell and T-cell function, reduce the effectiveness of phagocytes to kill organisms like Candida and cause atrophy of such important immune organs as the spleen and thymus.[2,3] The spleen and thymus glands are two structures in the body that are vital to helping the immune system fight off infections. Another study on the use of narcotics concluded that people with the potential for bacterial or viral infections should be cautioned against the use of narcotic medication.[4]

Narcotic medications, because of their potential immune-suppressing effect as well as their addictive properties, should be used as little as possible. Narcotic medications, as indicated above, can cause the shrinking of such important glands as the thymus and spleen.

A much more viable option than suppressing the pain with narcotic medications

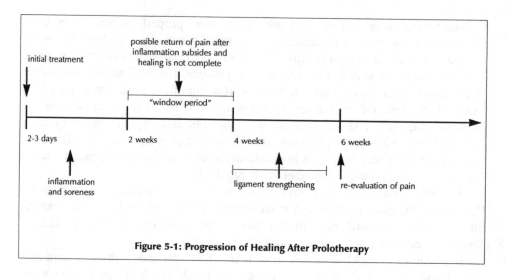

Figure 5-1: Progression of Healing After Prolotherapy

is to determine the root cause of the pain and correct it. Prolotherapy accomplishes this. If pain medicine is needed, Tylenol or Ultram can be used because they do not suppress inflammation. Anti-inflammatory medications, such as Motrin, Advil, or Voltaren, cannot be used because they suppress inflammation and block the beneficial effects of the Prolotherapy. Most people with chronic pain admit that they want to stop using pain medications. Often they say, "I just don't feel right being on those." Of course not. Would you feel "right" if your spleen and thymus were shrinking?

4. HOW MANY TREATMENTS ARE NECESSARY AND HOW OFTEN?

The anesthetic in the solution used during Prolotherapy sessions often provides immediate pain relief. The pain relief may continue after the effect of the anesthetic subsides due to the stabilizing of the treated joints because of the inflammation caused by the Prolotherapy injections. This pain relief normally continues for a few weeks after the first treatment.

Between the second and fourth weeks, the initial stabilization induced by the Prolotherapy subsides, and because the initial growth of ligament tissue is not complete, some of the original pain may return during this "window period" of healing. I recommend follow-up six weeks after each treatment to ensure an accurate assessment of results, avoiding an evaluation of a patient during the "window period." Prolotherapy is performed every six weeks because most ligaments heal over a six-week period.[5] **(Figure 5-1)**

As healing progresses, the quantity of injections required per treatment usually decreases. The pain generally continues to diminish with each treatment until it is completely eliminated. Four treatments are normally required to eliminate pain. Because everyone is unique, some people may only require one treatment while others will require as many as eight treatments. Rarely are more needed.

In some cases, patients will experience no pain relief after their first or second

Prolotherapy treatments. This does not mean the therapy is not working, rather it is an indication that the ligaments and tendons are not yet strong enough to stabilize the joints. The amount of collagen growth required for stabilization of the joint is different for each person. A patient who experiences pain relief at rest but not during activity requires further treatment to strengthen the area. If Prolotherapy treatments are continued, there is an excellent chance of achieving total pain relief with the resumption of all previous activities.

I tell all prospective patients who receive disability insurance or workman's compensation, are involved in a legal matter, or are on a leave of absence from work, that the ultimate goal of Prolotherapy treatments is to help the person return to normal function, including returning to work. In individuals who do not have a real desire to return to work or discontinue receiving disability insurance, Prolotherapy is not indicated. In such cases, the individuals do not possess a "real" desire to heal and Prolotherapy will not ease the pain as pain relief would be an admission that disability checks are no longer needed.

The above situation is a rarity in my office. The overwhelming majority of people suffering from chronic pain desire to find pain relief and return to work. A few of my patients have a phobia of needles. For those individuals, other Natural Medicine treatments are prescribed, but the results are significantly less dramatic than what is expected with Prolotherapy. Herbs and vitamins will not stabilize a chronically loose joint. Exercise will not stabilize a chronically loose joint. Prolotherapy is the one treatment that will. There is no substitute for Prolotherapy in regard to curing pain.

Patients who do not attain pain relief because of a phobia of needles or give up on Prolotherapy after one or two sessions because of slower than expected pain relief are needlessly living with chronic pain when a conservative, curative treatment is available. The number one reason for partial pain relief with Prolotherapy is not completing the full course of Prolotherapy sessions. It is important that the patient does not become disappointed if the pain is not relieved after one or two sessions, especially a patient who has been in pain for decades. I have had severe pain cases require only one treatment and relatively simple cases require six sessions.

Overcoming phobias and fears is difficult, but worthwhile and often produces the most happiness. My phobia was girls. In high school, I was often too scared to ask a girl for a date. There was one particular girl's picture I fell in love with when I was 12 years of age while looking through my year book at Jack Benny Junior High School in Waukegan, Illinois. It wasn't until after high school graduation that I was brave enough to call her. We talked and laughed for hours at Bevier Park in Waukegan, Illinois, on July 19, 1980. Seventeen years later, we are still talking and laughing. I'm sure glad that I had the courage to call her that day. My life would be pretty empty without my beautiful wife by my side. We must often overcome our fears to enjoy the true happiness that life offers.

5. IS PROLOTHERAPY COVERED BY INSURANCE?

Some insurance companies cover Prolotherapy while others do not. The usual

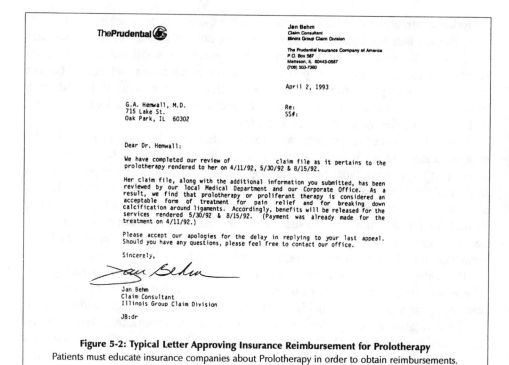

Figure 5-2: Typical Letter Approving Insurance Reimbursement for Prolotherapy
Patients must educate insurance companies about Prolotherapy in order to obtain reimbursements.

reason for denying coverage is that Prolotherapy is not a "usual and customary treatment." **(Figure 5-2)**

The Chicago Medical Society, a branch of the American Medical Society (AMA), reviewed a case for Aetna Life & Casualty Company and submitted the following on April 20, 1976 to Dr. Hemwall regarding their decision. "In response to the insurance carrier's request of whether your treatment [Prolotherapy] is an approved and appropriate method, the Subcommittee on Insurance Mediation has made a decision on the above entitled matter. On the basis of the information presented, it is the Committee's opinion that this procedure is an accepted procedure."[6] *(See Appendix F, Insurance Reimbursement Letters.)*

A few years later, the procedure was again reviewed by the Chicago Medical Society. In a letter dated November 1, 1979 to the Life Investors Insurance Company of America, the chairman of the Medical Practice Committee wrote, "It is the opinion of the Committee that, while the treatment does not enjoy widespread acceptance in medical circles, it is a well recognized procedure in veterinary medicine: animal models of disease and treatment form the basis for a great deal of medical knowledge and progress. It is significant to this Committee that Dr. Hemwall has performed this procedure on a great many people over an eighteen year period of time and our Society has never received a patient complaint on the procedure. It appears to us that this record speaks for successful treatment. We do not feel that either we, or an insurance carrier, are in a position to declare an uncommon, but apparently successful, procedure as an improper one. Because the method is not widely used does not mean that it is not compensable. A search of our records reveals that another Committee of our Society was presented with a similar question regarding 'Prolotherapy' (the previous reference) and they found it an accepted procedure and recommended payment of the physicians fees. We agree."[7]

The third time the Chicago Medical Society reviewed Prolotherapy was on November 5, 1987. Peter C. Pulos, M.D., Chairman of the Medical Practice Committee wrote this concerning Prolotherapy, "We understand that this procedure has been used by many medical and osteopathic physicians both in this country and in Europe. It is significant that Dr. Hemwall has performed this procedure on many people for almost 30 years and our Society has never received a complaint on the use of the procedure. It appears to the committee that this record speaks for successful treatment, and it is long past the stage where it is considered experimental. **...In light of our current review, it is the opinion of the Medical Practice Committee that the procedure of ligament injection, known as Prolotherapy, is a clinically accepted procedure and we recommend payment of the physicians fees by the insurance company."**[8] [Emphasis mine.]

The American Medical Association, of which the Chicago Medical Society is a local branch, is headquartered in Chicago. The Chicago Medical Society is one of the largest local branches of the American Medical Association, and the stamp of approval was given for Prolotherapy on three separate occasions over the last 20 years.

6. IF PROLOTHERAPY IS SO EFFECTIVE, WHY IS MY DOCTOR NOT AWARE OF IT?

Prolotherapy has been presented and taught for years by the American Association of Orthopedic Medicine, the American Board of Sclerotherapy, and The George S. Hackett Foundation. (*See Appendix D, George S. Hackett AMA Presentations.*) Presentations on Prolotherapy have been given at numerous medical conferences including the First and Second Interdisciplinary World Congresses on Low Back Pain sponsored by the University of California at San Diego, "Practical Approaches to Low Back Pain" sponsored by the University of Wisconsin Medical School, and most recently the New Frontiers in Pain 1996 meeting. In October 1996, at the national meeting of the American Academy of Physical Medicine and Rehabilitation, K. Dean Reeves, M.D., Ed Magaziner, M.D., and I presented a symposium on the treatment of chronic pain with Prolotherapy.

In addition to medical conferences, abundant references and research regarding Prolotherapy is available. The latest book on the different procedures used in Physical Medicine and Rehabilitation, *Physiatric Procedures*, contains a chapter devoted exclusively to Prolotherapy.[9] Dr. Reeves, in addition to writing that chapter, contributed an article on Prolotherapy in a recent issue of *Physical Medicine and Rehabilitation Clinics of North America*.[10] William Faber, D.O., and Thomas Dorman, M.D., have written numerous articles and have published several books devoted to the treatment of chronic pain with Prolotherapy.[11,12,13] Physicians such as these have done their best to spread the word about Prolotherapy, but it is still relatively unknown.

Instead of asking me why your doctor is not aware of Prolotherapy, give your doctor this book and ask him or her that question. Anyone involved in chronic pain management has the opportunity to learn about Prolotherapy.

7. WHY MAY PHYSICAL THERAPY, MASSAGE, AND CHIROPRACTIC MANIPULATION PROVIDE ONLY TEMPORARY RELIEF?

For the chronic pain patient, the source of the pain is most commonly due to ligament laxity. These therapies usually treat the symptoms and not the underlying cause. Physical therapy modalities such as TENS units, electrical stimulation units, massage, and ultrasound will decrease muscle spasm and permanently relieve pain if muscles are the source of the problem. The chronic pain patients' muscles are in spasm or are tense usually because the underlying joint is hypermobile, or loose, and the muscles contract in order to stabilize the joint. Chronic muscle tension and spasm is a sign that the underlying joints have ligament injury.

Manual manipulation is a very effective treatment for eliminating acute pain by realigning vertebral and bony structures. Temporary benefit after years of manipulation treatment is an indication that vertebral segments are weak because of lax ligaments. Continued manipulation will not strengthen vertebral segments. Weak vertebral ligaments are the cause of the malaligned vertebrae, known as subluxation.

The common source of chronic pain is loose joints, which is not resolved by manipulative treatment. However, any treatment that improves blood flow while undergoing Prolotherapy, such as massage, myofascial release, body work, ultrasound, and heat will enhance the body's response to Prolotherapy.

8. WHAT ENHANCES OR LIMITS LIGAMENT AND TENDON TISSUE HEALING?

There are many factors that are involved in a person's ability to heal after Prolotherapy. Age, obesity, hormones, nutrition, sleep, physical activity, medications, concurrent treatment regimes used, and infections are some of these factors. All of these have an effect on a person's immune function. Good immune function is needed for a person to adequately heal soft tissue injuries and respond well to Prolotherapy.

Prolotherapy initiates the growth of ligament and tendon tissue, but the body actually grows the tissue. If the body is deprived of the necessary building blocks to grow strong new tissue, the response to Prolotherapy will be reduced. Therefore all factors that decrease tendon and ligament growth should be increased before and during Prolotherapy to ensure complete healing. Prolotherapy's effectiveness and the body's ability to complete the healing process is different for each individual.
[14,15,16,17,18]

9. WHAT IS THE EFFECT OF AGE ON HEALING?

I frequently speak to retirement groups and am always amazed how few people truly enjoy retirement. My father-in-law retired about 12 years ago. He currently exercises three times a week, enjoys wonderful health, visits his children and grand-

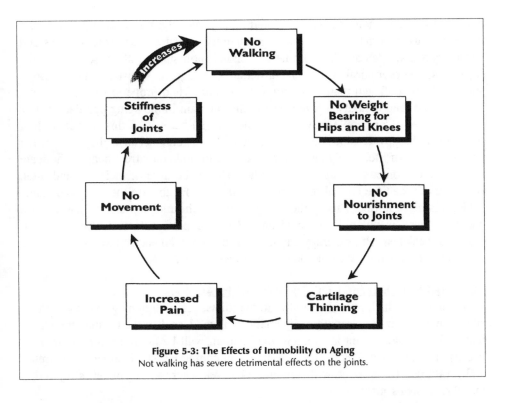

Figure 5-3: The Effects of Immobility on Aging
Not walking has severe detrimental effects on the joints.

children, and travels with his wife around the country. When my wife and I work at our charity clinic in southern Illinois, he uses his work experience as a chemist to perform all of the REAMS testing. He has far more energy than most younger folks at the clinic. This is how retirement should be for everyone!

What I have seen is usually the opposite. People's faces grimacing in pain when getting up from a chair, and a body that is bent over a walker when ambulating is more typical. Unfortunately, people are forced to use canes, walkers, or wheel-chairs for transportation. Some reside in nursing homes because of their ill health. I would prefer my father-in-law's type of retirement.

I am also amazed at how few people seek out Prolotherapy treatments after learning that relief from their pain is possible. It appears that the feeling among the aged is that pain is just a normal part of the aging process. There is no honor in needlessly suffering from pain.

Losing the ability to be mobile and active is possibly the worst thing that can happen to people as they age. Activity truly keeps the blood flowing. Joints like the hips and knees depend on walking and weight-bearing activities to provide nourish-ment to the joint cartilage. No walking, no nourishment. No nourishment, no carti-lage. No cartilage, no movement. Walking keeps people alive and keeps the body functioning. If stiffness sets in, the grave may follow. **(Figure 5-3)**

Because most bodily functions decline with age, the ability to heal an injury and the immune system response are slower. With age, the ligament and tendon tissue contain less water, noncollagenous protein, and proteoglycans. Proteoglycans are a proteinaceous material containing a large quantity of water. The proteoglycans and subcomponents, such as glucosamine and chondroitin sulfate, allow structures like ligaments, intervertebral discs, and articular cartilage to withstand intense pressure.[19,20,21] The collagen matrix becomes disorganized and prone to injury. Chronic ligament and tendon laxity is a reason for chronic pain in the aging population. For these reasons, older people may respond slower and because of this slower healing more Prolotherapy sessions may be needed. Teenagers, because they are in the growing phase of life, rarely need more than one Prolotherapy treatment to eliminate chronic pain. Someone in their 90s will heal slower because of their age and often require more than the typical four Prolotherapy sessions to cure their chronic pain.

Pain is not a normal part of the aging process. Chronic pain always has a cause and that cause is not old age syndrome. Chronic pain is almost always due to ligament weakness. Prolotherapy can help strengthen ligaments at any age and is the treatment of choice for chronic pain, regardless of age.

10. WHAT IS THE EFFECT OF OBESITY ON HEALING?

Ligaments, which provide stability to the joints, resist stretching (have good tensile strength). Tensile strength of ligaments is much less than the tensile strength of bone. Thus, when a joint is stressed, the ligament will be injured prior to the bone because it is the weak link of the bone-ligament complex.[22] The ligament will stretch and sprain before the bone will fracture. The area where the ligament is injured is the fibro-osseous junction.

The strength of the ligament required to maintain the stability of the joint depends directly on the pressure applied. The heavier the force applied to the joint, the stronger the ligament must be to hold the joint in place. A tackle by Dick Butkus, former middle linebacker of the Chicago Bears, requires ligaments to withstand more pressure in order to maintain knee stability than being tackled by me. This explains why overweight people, exhibiting a positive "basketball-belly sign," are prone to chronic pain and impaired healing. The excess weight places increased pressure on the ligaments, especially in the lower back, hip, and knee areas. These ligaments stretch and weaken and begin the process known as osteoarthritis.

Weight loss is effective for decreasing the pain of osteoarthritis and chronic ligament and tendon weakness because it diminishes the stress on the joints. Stabilization and movement of the joint requires less work by the ligaments and tendons, resulting in reduced pain.

11. DO HORMONES PLAY A ROLE IN HEALING?

The endocrine system produces and secretes hormones for the body, including adrenal hormones such as cortisol, thyroid hormones, growth hormone, melatonin, prostaglandins, and insulin. Hormones such as testosterone, cortisol, and thyroxine regulate the growth of tissue. An inadequate endocrine system will propagate ligament and tendon weakness. Soft tissue healing of ligaments and tendons will be compromised if any of these hormones are deficient.[23,24,25] Hormone levels also naturally decrease with age. Therefore, these hormones may need to be supplemented in order to ensure complete healing.

To be evaluated for hormone deficiencies and the use of natural hormones, an evaluation by a Natural Medicine physician should be considered. (*To locate a Natural Medicine physician near you, contact the organizations listed in Appendix C, Natural Medicine Resources.*)

12. WHAT IS THE ROLE OF NUTRITION IN HEALING?

Nutritional deficiencies are epidemic in modern society affecting both overall health and the healing of ligaments and tendons. Ligaments and tendons consist of water, proteoglycans, and collagen. Collagen represents 70 to 90 percent of the weight of connective tissues and is the most abundant protein in the human body, approximately 30 percent of total proteins, and six percent of human body weight.

Collagen synthesis requires specific nutrients including iron, copper, manganese, calcium, zinc, vitamin C, and various amino acids.[26] Proteoglycan synthesis requires the coordination of protein, carbohydrate polymer, and collagen synthesis, along with trace minerals such as manganese, copper, and zinc. Proper nutrition is an essential factor in soft tissue healing. A diet lacking in adequate nutrients such as vitamin A, vitamin C, zinc, and protein will hinder the healing process and the formation of collagen tissue. For these reasons, everyone should take a good multivitamin and mineral supplement.

It is also important that we eat an appropriate diet for our metabolism and take vitamins according to our metabolic type. (*See Appendix A, Nutrition and Chronic Pain, to learn more about Metabolic Typing.*) To assist healing after Prolotherapy, I recommend a nutritional supplement called Ortho Prolo Max which contains specific nutrients that are needed in soft tissue healing. (*See Appendix C, Natural Medicine Resources, for information on how to obtain Ortho Prolo Max.*)

Water is the most necessary nutrient in the body. The human body is composed of 25 percent solid matter and 75 percent water. Many of the supporting structures of the body, including the articular cartilage surfaces of joints and the intervertebral discs, contain a significant amount of water. Seventy-five percent of the weight of the upper part of the body is supported by the water volume stored in the disc core.[27] Inadequate intake of water may lead to inadequate fluid support to these areas, resulting in weakened structures that may produce chronic pain. In order to determine the amount of water you should drink daily, divide your body weight in pounds by two. This equals the amount of water you should drink in ounces per day. For example, a 150 pound man should drink 75 ounces of distilled, filtered water per day.

13. WHAT IS THE ROLE OF SLEEP IN HEALING?

Chronic pain patients are often prescribed anti-depressant medications like Elavil to aid sleep. These medicines provide some temporary pain relief and aid sleep. However, chronic pain is not due to an Elavil or other pharmaceutical drug deficiency. Chronic pain has a cause. Until the etiology is determined and treated, all therapeutic modalities will provide only temporary relief. Prolotherapy injections

	PAIN-FREE	**CHRONIC PAIN**
Night Cortisol Levels	Low	High
State of Mind at Bedtime	Restful	Restless
End Result	Sleep	Insomnia

Figure 5-4: Effect of Chronic Pain on Cortisol Levels and Sleep
Chronic pain leads to high cortisol levels at bedtime which results in an awake state of mind and chronic insomnia.

to strengthen the ligament and tendon attachments to bone cause permanent healing.

Chronic pain and chronic insomnia go hand in hand. The adrenal gland secretion of the hormone cortisol normally decreases at night and the pineal gland secretion of melatonin increases, thereby enabling sleep. Unfortunately, the chronic pain patient's secretion of cortisol does not decline because chronic pain is seen by the body as stress, thereby stimulating the adrenal gland, which reacts to stress, to produce cortisol. This results in chronic insomnia. **(Figure 5-4)** The secretion of cortisol will stop only when the chronic pain is relieved. Chronic insomnia increases chronic pain. Prolotherapy breaks this cycle. Pain relief leads to a good night's sleep.

Sleep is vital to health maintenance. Sleep stimulates the anterior pituitary to produce growth hormone. Growth hormone is one of the main anabolic, meaning to grow or repair, hormones in the body whose job is to repair the damage done to the body during the day. Every day, soft tissues including ligaments and tendons are damaged. It is vital to obtain deep stages of sleep, as during this time growth hormone is secreted.

Without deep stages of sleep, inadequate growth hormone is secreted and soft tissue healing is inadequate. **(Figure 5-5)** Growth hormone levels also appear to be increased with exercise and amino acid supplementation with ornithine, arginine, or glutamine.[28,29]

A natural way to increase sleep and improve deep sleep is aerobic exercise like cycling, walking, or rebounding. Melatonin, L-Tryptophan (an amino acid) valerian root, and gamma hydroxybutyrate are also beneficial natural sleep aids.

14. WHAT IS THE ROLE OF PHYSICAL ACTIVITY IN HEALING?

Exercise is currently the traditional treatment of choice for chronic pain. Chronic pain patients often experience an exacerbation of their pain when exercising. This is an indication that ligament laxity is the cause of the pain. Ligament laxity generally causes pain when the joint is stressed, which occurs with activity. The proper

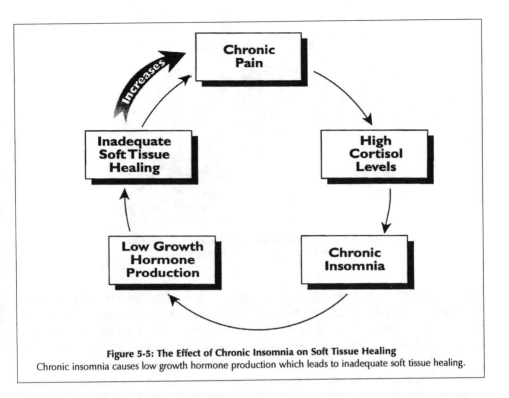

Figure 5-5: The Effect of Chronic Insomnia on Soft Tissue Healing
Chronic insomnia causes low growth hormone production which leads to inadequate soft tissue healing.

treatment is not to "work through the pain," but to correct the source of the pain. The main function of exercise is to strengthen muscle, not to grow ligament tissue.

Aggressive exercise may worsen ligament injury and is not recommended until Prolotherapy has strengthened the joint sufficiently to provide pain relief. A good rule-of-thumb is if doing something hurts, don't do it. Doctors are smart aren't they? Once healing begins and the pain has decreased, dynamic range-of-motion exercises like walking, cycling, and swimming are more helpful than static-resistive exercises like weight-lifting.[30] A more formal exercise program is necessary after the ligaments strengthen and the joint stabilizes. This exercise program will strengthen the muscles around the joint and increase the flexibility of the muscles which protect the joint from reinjury.

15. SHOULD I IMMOBILIZE THE INJURED AREA?

Immobilization, also known as stress deprivation, is extremely detrimental to the body's joints and ligaments. Immobilization causes the following changes to occur inside joints: 1) proliferation of fatty connective tissue within the joint, 2) cartilage damage and necrosis, 3) scar tissue formation and articular cartilage tears, 4) increased randomness of the collagen fibers within the ligaments and connective tissues, and 5) ligament weakening with a decreased resistance to stretch.[31,32,33]

A study performed on animals revealed that after several weeks of immobilization, the strength of the ligament tissue was reduced to about one-third of normal.[34,35,36,37]

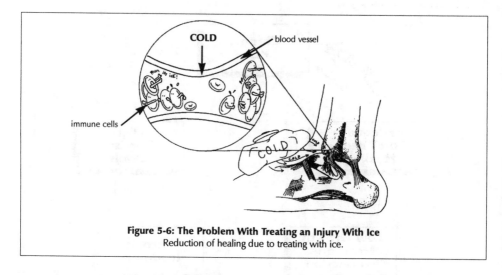

Figure 5-6: The Problem With Treating an Injury With Ice
Reduction of healing due to treating with ice.

Immobilization also significantly decreases the strength of the fibro-osseous junction, the bone-ligament interface.[38] Eight weeks of immobilization produced a 39 percent decrease in the strength of the fibro-osseous junction of the anterior cruciate ligament of the knee.[39,40] Other researchers have shown that even partial immobilization (restricted activity) has similar deleterious effects on ligament insertion sites.[41]

Immobility causes decreased water content, decreased proteoglycans, increased collagen turnover, and a dramatic alteration in the type of collagen cross-linking of the ligaments producing a weak ligament.[42,43] Immobility is one of the primary reasons ligaments heal inadequately after an injury.

Unfortunately, the standard treatment for a tendon strain or ligament sprain is **R**est, **I**ce, **C**ompression, and **E**levation, also known as RICE. Any emergency room or sports medicine book will recommend this same course of treatment. I recently received a newsletter from the local hospital of which I am on staff which recommended the RICE treatment for an acute soft tissue injury of a ligament or tendon. This treatment is provided because the pain is relieved in the short-term. However, research reveals that the RICE treatment actually impairs healing and contributes to chronic ligament and tendon relaxation. Any treatment that impairs soft tissue healing increases the risk of incomplete ligament and tendon repair and predisposes the structure to future injury and becoming a source of chronic pain.

16. SHOULD I PUT ICE ON MY INJURY?

As a result of immobilization (rest), ice, compression, and elevation blood flow is decreased, resulting in reduced immune cell production necessary to remove the debris from the injury site. This produces formation of weak ligament and tendon tissue. **(Figure 5-6)** Swelling is the physical manifestation of inflammation. Swelling is evidence that the body is working to heal itself. Use of ice will obviously prevent the body from doing its work. Ice treatment has many harmful effects. It has been shown that as little as five minutes of icing a knee can decrease both blood flow to the soft tissues and skeletal metabolism.[44] Icing an area for 25 minutes decreases blood flow and skeletal metabolism another 400 percent. Healing is hindered by a decrease in blood flow and metabolism to the area. Icing increases the chance of incomplete healing by decreasing blood flow to the injured ligaments and tendons. This increases the chance of re-injury or the development of chronic pain.

17. IS PROLOTHERAPY USEFUL FOR ACUTE INJURIES?

If inflammation is so beneficial, why not use Prolotherapy for the treatment of an acute injury? Prolotherapy is beneficial and will speed the recovery process of an acute injury. However, I always recommend the first treatment be the most conservative one. A more conservative approach to treating acute injuries to ligaments and tendons is Movement, Exercise, Analgesics, and Treatment, also known as MEAT. While immobility is detrimental to soft tissue healing, movement is beneficial.[45] Movement and gentle range-of-motion exercises improve blood flow to the area, removing debris. Heat also increases blood flow so this is recommended after an acute injury. If movement of the joint is painful, then isometric exercises should be performed. Isometric exercising involves contracting a muscle without movement of the affected joint. An example of this is a handshake. Both parties squeeze, creating a muscle contraction without joint movement.

Natural analgesics or pain relievers that are not synthetic anti-inflammatories may be used. Natural substances such as the enzymes bromelain, Trypsin, and Papain aid soft tissue healing by reducing the viscosity of extracellular fluid. This increases nutrient and waste transport from the injured site, reducing swelling or edema.[46] A narcotic such as codeine may be prescribed short term for an extremely painful acute injury. Narcotics are wonderful pain relievers and do not interfere with the natural healing mechanisms of the body, if used in the short-term. Your body produces its own narcotics, called endorphins, which work to reduce pain from an acute injury. Other options for pain control include Tylenol or Ultram. As previously mentioned, these can be used as they relieve pain but do not decrease inflammation.

The "T" in MEAT stands for specific Treatments that increase blood flow and immune cell migration to the damaged area which will aid in ligament and tendon healing. Treatments such as physical therapy, massage, chiropractic care, ultrasound, myofascial release, and electrical stimulation all improve blood flow and assist soft tissue healing. **(Figure 5-7)**

If circumstances are such that time is a factor, some Prolotherapy physicians will use Prolotherapy as an initial treatment for acute pain. Rodney Van Pelt, M.D., utilizes Prolotherapy in the management of acute sports injury. An athlete who would normally wait two to three months for an acute injury to heal may heal in only two to three weeks if given Prolotherapy. Dr. Van Pelt has seen this increased speed of recovery in a multitude of sports injuries including ACL (anterior cruciate ligament) sprains of the knee. The late David Brewer, M.D., who was an obstetrician and gynecologist, used Prolotherapy in the treatment of low back pain of pregnancy. This safe and effective treatment is extremely helpful in relieving the low back pain experienced during and after pregnancy.

RICE versus MEAT

	RICE	MEAT
Immune System Response	Decreased	Increased
Blood Flow to Injured Area	Decreased	Increased
Collagen Formation	Hindered	Encouraged
Speed of Recovery	Delayed (Lengthened)	Hastened (Shortened)
Range of Motion of Joint	Decreased	Increased
Complete Healing	Decreased	Increased

Figure 5-7: RICE versus MEAT
The RICE protocol hampers soft tissue healing whereas MEAT encourages healing.

18. CAN I TAKE ANTI-INFLAMMATORY AGENTS?

Anti-inflammatory medicines, like Motrin, Advil, aspirin, Clinoril, Volteran, Prednisone, and Cortisone, all inhibit the healing process of soft tissues. The long-term detrimental effects far outweigh the temporary positive effect of decreased pain. Aspirin does have a beneficial effect on the heart, but a detrimental effect on soft tissue healing. When a ligament or tendon is injured, prostaglandins are released which initiate vasodilation in noninjured blood vessels. This enables healthy blood vessels to increase blood flow and immune cell flow to the injured area to begin the repair process. The use of anti-inflammatories inhibits the release of prostaglandins thus ultimately decreasing the blood flow to the injured area.[47]

As previously stated, nonsteroidal anti-inflammatory drugs (NSAIDs) have been shown to produce short-term pain benefit but leave long-term loss of function.[48] NSAIDs also inhibit proteoglycan synthesis, a component of ligament and cartilage tissue. Proteoglycans are essential for the elasticity and compressive stiffness of articular cartilage and suppression of their synthesis has significant adverse effects on the joint.[49,50,51]

NSAID prescription for acute soft tissue injury is considered standard practice. The administration of NSAIDs, in combination with the RICE treatment, nearly eliminates the body's ability to heal. Is it any wonder so many people live with chronic pain? In my opinion, the current medical treatment for acute soft tissue injuries is contributing to this epidemic.

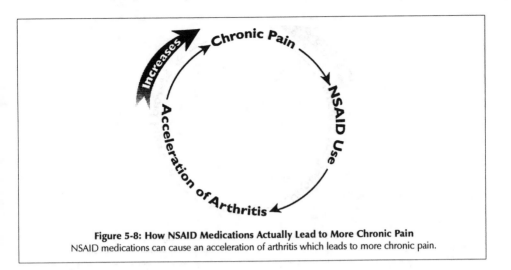

Figure 5-8: How NSAID Medications Actually Lead to More Chronic Pain
NSAID medications can cause an acceleration of arthritis which leads to more chronic pain.

NSAIDs are the mainstay treatment for acute ligament and tendon injuries, yet efficacy in their usefulness is lacking.[52] Worse yet is the long-term use by people with chronic pain. Studies in the use of NSAIDs for chronic hip pain revealed an acceleration of arthritis in the people taking NSAIDs.[53,54,55]

In one study, NSAID use was associated with progressive formation of multiple small acetabular and femoral subcortical cysts and subchondral bone thinning. In this study, 84 percent of the people who had progressive arthritis were long-term NSAID users. The conclusion of the study was "this highly significant association between NSAID use and acetabular destruction gives cause for concern."[56] As it should, acetabular destruction, femoral subcortical cysts, and subchondral bone thinning are all signs that the NSAIDs were causing arthritis to form more quickly. This is one explanation why people taking Motrin, Advil, Voltaren, or any other NSAID will likely require more medicine to decrease their pain. Eventually the medicine does not stop the pain because the arthritis process is actually accelerating while taking the medicine. **(Figure 5-8)**

The end result of taking NSAIDs for pain relief is an arthritic joint. How many times has Motrin or any other NSAID cured a person of his or her pain? Prolotherapy eliminates the cause of chronic pain and often cures the person's pain. Even long-term aspirin use has been associated with accelerating hip damage from arthritis.[57] When comparing the long-term use of Indomethacin in the treatment of osteoarthritis of the hip it was clearly shown that the disease progressed more frequently and the destruction within the hip joint was more severe with drug use than without.[58]

For women of child-bearing age who want to have children but have pain, Prolotherapy is a better choice for another reason.[59] NSAIDs have caused concern that they may be associated with an increase rate of infertility in females because they delay the egg from being released. NSAIDs are truly anti-inflammatory in their mechanism of action. Since all tissues heal by inflammation, one can see why long-

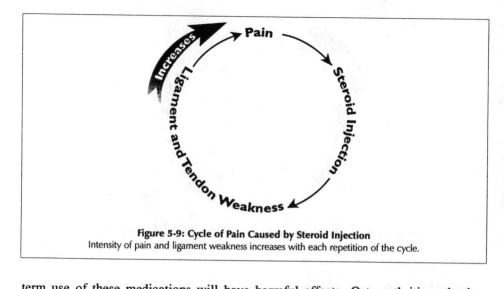

Figure 5-9: Cycle of Pain Caused by Steroid Injection
Intensity of pain and ligament weakness increases with each repetition of the cycle.

term use of these medications will have harmful effects. Osteoarthritis and other chronic pain disorders are not an Indomethacin or other NSAID deficiency. This is why the use of these drugs will never cure any disease. Their chronic long-term use will not cure, and will hamper soft tissue healing and accelerate the arthritic process.

Prolotherapy, because it stimulates inflammation, helps the body heal itself. Prolotherapy stops the arthritic process and helps eliminate the person's chronic pain, often permanently. NSAIDs should not be taken while undergoing Prolotherapy because they inhibit the inflammation caused by the treatment. For that matter, anyone with chronic pain should seriously consider stopping NSAIDs and starting Prolotherapy.

19. WHAT ABOUT STEROID INJECTIONS?

The next assault to the already weakened ligament and tendon tissue after RICE and NSAID treatments is the steroid injection. The unfortunate person who has been subjected to RICE and NSAID treatments will likely be offered a steroid injection for the pain which has now become chronic. The RICE- and NSAID-weakened ligament and tendon will be further attacked by each subsequent steroid injection. A cyclical pattern of injury, improper treatment, further injury, and ultimately, chronic pain, emerges. This leads to further weakness in the tissue and the cycle repeats itself. **(Figure 5-9)**

Corticosteroids, such as Cortisone and Prednisone, have an adverse effect on bone and soft tissue healing. Corticosteroids inactivate vitamin D, limiting calcium absorption by the gastrointestinal tract and increasing urinary excretion of calcium. Bone also shows a decrease in calcium uptake, ultimately leading to weakness at the fibro-osseous junction. Corticosteroids also inhibit the release of growth hormone which further decreases soft tissue and bone repair. Ultimately, corticosteroids lead to a decrease in bone, ligament, and tendon strength.[60,61,62,63,64,65]

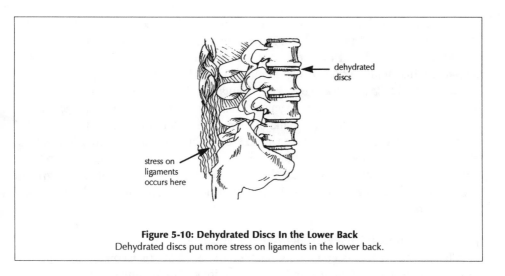

Figure 5-10: Dehydrated Discs In the Lower Back
Dehydrated discs put more stress on ligaments in the lower back.

Corticosteroids inhibit the synthesis of proteins, collagen, and proteoglycans in articular cartilage, by inhibiting chondrocyte production, the cells that comprise the articular cartilage. The net catabolic effect (weakening) of corticosteroids is inhibition of fibroblast production of collagen, ground substance, and angiogenesis (new blood vessel formation). The result is weakened synovial joints, supporting structures, and ligaments and tendons. This weakness increases pain and the increased pain leads to more steroid injections. Corticosteroids should not be used as a treatment for chronic pain due to ligament and tendon weakness. The treatment of choice for such conditions is Prolotherapy.

20. WHAT IS pH AND HOW DOES IT AFFECT HEALING?

I utilize a simple diagnostic testing procedure known as Metabolic Typing to determine a person's underlying physiology.[66,67] (*See Appendix A, Nutrition and Chronic Pain, for more information on Metabolic Typing.*) The test consists of, among other things, determining blood, urine, and saliva pH. The tests consistently reveal that chronic pain patients suffer from chronic dehydration. Chronic dehydration produces a reduction in shock absorbing capabilities of the intervertebral discs and articular cartilage, placing additional stress on the ligaments to stabilize the joints. The end result is ligament laxity, injury, and resultant chronic pain. **(Figure 5-10)** It is very important for the person in chronic pain to drink six to eight glasses of purified water per day.

I have found that a significant number of chronic pain patients have a lower than normal venous blood plasma pH.[68] A person with low venous plasma pH has what is termed acid blood. Acid blood is typically dark in color due to low oxygen content. Oxygen is the food that allows the body to extract and store energy from the blood. A low oxygen content in the blood compromises healing capabilities.

The treatment for acid blood is to consume foods and supplements which neutralize the blood pH. This is accomplished by consuming items which are alkaline and reducing the intake of acidic items. Caffeine, sugar, wheat, citrus fruits, soda pop, and potatoes should be avoided, whereas protein and vegetables should be the majority of the meal. Supplements such as green algae or alfalfa also help neutralize acidic blood. A diet similar to that discussed by Barry Sears, Ph.D. in the book *The Zone* works very well.[69] Nuts, seeds, brown rice, or soy products are good sources of protein if a vegetarian diet is preferred. People with acid blood are typically carbohydrate addicts and consume very little protein. Protein is needed in the diet because collagen, which makes up ligaments and tendons, is the most abundant protein in the body. Collagen is the building block for ligament and tendon tissue. A healthy diet with adequate amounts of protein for soft tissue growth is essential for healing ligament and tendon injuries. (*See Appendix A, Nutrition and Chronic Pain.*)

21. DOES CHRONIC INFECTION AFFECT HEALING?

Chronic pain patients commonly possess a myriad of other conditions including diabetes, allergies, and fungal and sinus infections. The immune system's primary function is to sustain life. If chronic sinus or fungal infection exists, the immune system will preferentially fight these conditions versus healing a ligament or tendon injury. Controlling all infections, allergies, or other chronic health problems is essential to healing chronic ligament or tendon injury. I prefer to use natural treatments like garlic, echinacea, tea tree oil, and goldenseal to fight infections. In regard to allergies, I recommend facial dipping which cleanses the nose. The nose is a filter and should be cleansed periodically. Facial dipping involves dipping the face in an iodine-salt-water mixture and breathing it up into the nostrils. It works great! Natural botanicals such as stinging nettles, curcumin, and quercetin also decrease allergic symptoms. (*See Appendix C, Natural Medicine Resources.*) This is one of the reasons that anyone with chronic pain should see a Prolotherapist, as most Prolotherapists also practice Natural Medicine.

22. WHAT IS THE ROLE OF IMMUNE FUNCTION IN HEALING?

All of the above reasons for inadequate soft tissue healing have one thing in common, they all lead to suboptimal immune function. Immune function declines with age, and endocrine or nutritional inadequacies. Immobility, RICE, NSAIDs, infections, allergies, acid blood, and poor tissue oxygenation all cause a decline in the immune response. This poor immune response causes poor ligament and tissue healing, resulting in chronic pain. Chronic pain may lead to immobility and subsequent use of NSAIDs, which leads to insomnia and depression, which causes some people to eat "lousy" (or at least gives them an excuse), which can lead to acid blood and poor tissue oxygenation, producing further tissue and tendon weakness. There is only one thing that can break this cycle: Prolotherapy.

If these above issues are addressed, a person who has chronic pain as a result of ligament or tendon injury has an excellent prognosis for complete healing with Prolotherapy.

CHAPTER 6

Prolotherapy, Inflammation, and Healing: What's the Connection?

D uring my fourth year of medical school, on a dermatology rotation with four other medical students, I had the opportunity to train under Gary Solomon, M.D., one of the most respected dermatologists in the country. Dr. Solomon told us he was going to give us the secret to understanding human disease. If we knew the secret we would be leaps and bounds ahead of our colleagues and be masterful clinicians. I couldn't wait!

When that day finally arrived, Dr. Solomon explained that **inflammation** was the most important concept to understanding health and healing, especially in regard to the etiology and treatment of human ailments. Most clinicians do not understand inflammation, he said.

Inflammation?! E-Gads! Everyone knows about inflammation, I reasoned. I dismissed his comments and left disappointed. Years later when I learned about Prolotherapy, I realized Dr. Solomon had been right. Inflammation is the mechanism by which the body heals, regardless of the illness.

AN OLYMPIC-SIZE EXAMPLE

Kerri Strug became the heroine of the 1996 Summer Olympics by "sticking" her final vault to secure a gold medal for the American team in women's gymnastics. The most dramatic aspect of this vault was that she flew through the air and landed on a badly sprained ankle. As she lay wincing in pain after her heroic vault, she was mauled by medical personnel.

Unfortunately, she was observed throughout the rest of the Olympics with her ankle wrapped and her foot elevated. "What will happen to Kerri Strug? Will she finish the competition?" viewers wondered. "Will she be left with a weak ankle? Will she have chronic pain?" If the medical treatment she received at the Olympics is any indication, she will be anti-inflaming her pain to stay.

Kerri Strug suffered a ligament sprain. Ligaments are the supporting structures of the musculoskeletal system that connect the bones to each other. A stretched and weakened ligament is defined as a sprain.

Immediately after her ligament injury, Kerri Strug was given the currently accepted mode of treatment known as RICE. This treatment is prescribed by most physicians, athletic trainers, physical therapists, and chiropractors for an acute injury of a ligament or tendon. The treatment consists of **R**est, **I**ce, **C**ompression,

RICE versus MEAT

Modality	Result	Modality	Result
Rest	decreased joint nutrition	Mobility	increased joint nutrition
Ice	decreased blood flow	Exercise	increased blood flow
Compression	decreased pain control	Analgesic	increased pain control
Elevation	incomplete healing	Treatment	complete healing

Figure 6-1: RICE versus MEAT
The RICE treatment leads to incomplete healing of soft tissue whereas MEAT encourages complete healing.

and Elevation in order to immobilize the joint and decrease the swelling. The short-term result of this treatment is a reduction in pain. For the treatment of soft tissue injury, however, the RICE treatment decreases blood flow preventing immune cells from getting to the injured area. This impairs the healing process, causes greater pain long-term, and increases the chance of incomplete healing of the injured ligament. **(Figure 6-1)**

WHERE COMPLETE HEALING BEGINS

All human ailments, including ligament and tendon injury, involve inflammation. Inflammation is defined as the reaction of vascularized living tissue to local injury.[1] The first stage of inflammation is the actual injury. Inflammation is the body's reaction to a local injury. Healing an injured area is dependent on the blood supplying inflammatory cells to repair the damaged tissue, which explains why vascularized living tissue is crucial to the repair of any injured area. Vascularization refers to the blood supply to an area. Poor blood flow proportionately reduces healing.

Chronically weak ligaments and tendons are a result of inadequate repair following an injury and occur because of poor blood supply to the area where ligaments and tendons attach to the bone, the fibro-osseous junction.[2,3,4] **(Figure 6-2)** Due to the poor blood supply, the immune cells necessary to repair the affected area cannot reach the injury. Inadequate healing is the result. Nonsteroidal anti-inflammatory drugs (NSAIDs) and ice treatments decrease the blood flow even further thus hampering the body's capability to heal the injured tissue.

Healing of an injured tissue, such as a ligament, progresses through a series of stages: inflammatory, fibroblastic, and maturation.[5,6,7] The inflammatory stage is characterized by an increase in blood flow transporting healing immune cells to the area, often resulting in painful swelling. Swelling tells the body, especially the brain, that an area of the body has been injured. The immune system is activated to send immune cells, called polymorphonuclear cells, also known as polys, to the

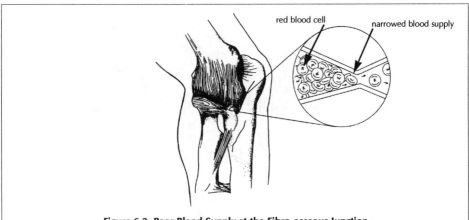

Figure 6-2: Poor Blood Supply at the Fibro-osseous Junction
The fibro-osseous junction normally has poor blood supply compared to other structures such as muscles.

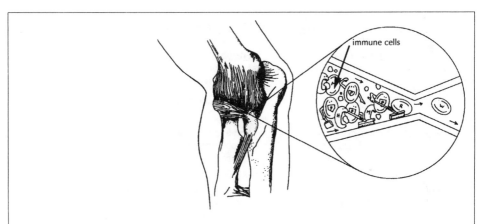

Figure 6-3: Immune System Activity at the Fibro-osseous Junction Immediately After an Injury
Responding to an injury, the immune system activates to remove debris.

injured area and remove the debris. **(Figure 6-3)** Other immune cells including the monocytes, histocytes, and macrophage cells assist in the cleanup. The macrophages and polys begin the process of phagocytosis, also called dinner, whereby they engulf and subsequently destroy debris and any other foreign matter in the body.

A day or two after the initial injury, the fibroblastic stage of healing begins. The body forms new blood vessels, a process called angiogenesis, because of factors released by the macrophage cells. Fibroblasts are formed from local cells or other immune cells in the blood. They are the carpenters of the body which form new collagen tissue, the building blocks of ligaments and tendons. **(Figure 6-4)** Collagen is responsible for the strength of the ligament and tendon. The fibroblastic stage continues for approximately six weeks after the injury. Consequently, Prolotherapy treatments are administered every six weeks, allowing maximal time for ligament

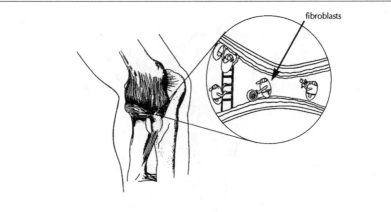

Figure 6-4: Immune System Growing Tissue at the Fibro-osseous Junction
Fibroblasts forming new collagen tissue which makes the ligament and tendon strong.

THREE STAGES OF HEALING

	Inflammation	**Fibroblastic**	**Maturation**
Effect on Blood	Increased blood flow.	Formation of new blood vessels.	New blood vessels mature.
Symptoms	Swelling and pain increase.	Swelling and pain subside.	If tissue is strong, pain subsides.
Physiology	Immune cells called macrophages remove damaged tissue.	Immune cells called fibroblasts form new collagen.	Increased density and diameter of collagen fibers occur if healing is not hindered.
Length of Time	Immediate response occurs for first week.	Begins at day 2 or 3 after injury and continues for 6 weeks.	Continues from day 42 until 18 months after injury.

Figure 6-5: Three Stages of Healing After Soft Tissue Injury

and tendon growth.[8]

The maturation phase of healing begins after the fibroblastic stage and may continue for 18 months after an injury. During this time the collagen fibers increase in density and diameter, resulting in increased strength. **(Figure 6-5)**

Anything that decreases inflammation is detrimental to the healing process of soft tissue injury. NSAIDs, for example, should only be prescribed when inflammation is the **cause** of the problem. In the case of soft tissue injury, inflammation is the **cure** for the problem. Prolotherapy injections stimulate ligament and tendon tissue growth, which only occurs through the process of inflammation. Dr. Solomon was indeed right. Inflammation is the key to the treatment of human ailments. Those who suffer from chronic pain have a choice: Anti-inflame the pain to stay or inflame your pain away with Prolotherapy.

CHAPTER 7

Prolo Your Back Pain Away

Baseball has its original iron man, Lou Gehrig and more recently Cal Ripken, but hockey's iron man will always be Stan Mikita of the Chicago Blackhawks. For 22 seasons, Stan dazzled hockey fans. His hockey career extended over four decades, from 1958 to 1980, during which time he amassed 1,467 total points, played in 18 playoff series, and was a member of the 1961 Stanley Cup championship team. Stan Mikita is truly an iron man.

But Stan did not feel like an iron man six weeks before the 1971-72 training camp. He had such excruciating back pain that he could not even get out of bed. Stan had learned to deal with constant back pain since injuring his back during a game in the 1960s. He had sought treatment from the Mayo Clinic and some of the best sports clinics and rehabilitation specialists without success.

"I knew something had to be done. I couldn't get out of bed," Stan said. "I had heard about Dr. Hemwall's Prolotherapy treatments and decided to give it a try." Gustav A. Hemwall, M.D., the world's most experienced Prolotherapist, treated Stan's lower back twice in three weeks. Aggressive treatment was given because Stan had to report to training camp.

"The results were unbelievable!" Stan exclaimed. "For the last eight years of my career I was completely pain free. I would say Prolotherapy definitely helped prolong my career." In 1983, Stan was elected to the National Hockey League Hall of Fame.

LIMITATIONS OF MRI AND CAT SCANS

Most medical physicians rely too heavily on diagnostic tests, especially for low back problems. Consequently, many who suffer from low back pain do not find relief. The typical scenario is as follows: A person complains to a physician about low back pain that radiates down the leg. The physician orders X-rays and a CAT or MRI scan. The MRI scan reveals an abnormality in the disc such as a herniated, bulging, or degenerated disc. Unfortunately for the patient, this finding usually has nothing to do with the pain. As discussed in Chapter Two, 50 percent of people over age 40 who are asymptomatic have such findings on a CAT scan.

In the 1980s, modern medicine developed another high-tech diagnostic tool to look at vertebrae, nerves, and discs on film—the MRI scan. Again, the same types of abnormalities were found in the vertebral discs and bones. People were subjected to various treatments and surgeries for these "abnormalities" in the hopes of curing their pain.

Very few people were cured. But all received hefty bills for the tests and surgeries.

Ten years of using MRI technology passed before research was conducted on the MRI findings of the lower back of people who had no pain symptoms.[1,2] Scott Boden, M.D., found that nearly 100 percent of the people he tested who were over 60 years of age with no symptoms had abnormal findings in their lumbar spines (lower back) on MRI scans. Thirty-six percent had herniated discs and all but one had degeneration or bulging of a disc in at least one lumbar level. In the age group of 20 to 39, 35 percent had degeneration or bulging of a disc in at least one lumbar level.[3]

In a study published in *The New England Journal of Medicine* in 1994, Maureen Jensen, M.D., and associates, studied MRI scans of the lumbar spine in 98 asymptomatic people. Only 36 percent had a normal scan, 64 percent had abnormal findings overall, and 38 percent had abnormal findings in more than one lumbar vertebral level. The conclusion was "because bulges and protrusions on MRI scans in people with low back pain or even radiculopathy may be coincidental, a patient's clinical situation must be carefully evaluated in conjunction with the results of MRI studies."[4] In other words, physicians should begin listening with their ears and poking with their thumbs! X-ray studies should never take the place of a good history and physical examination. Unfortunately for many, X-ray findings have nothing to do with their pain.

DIAGNOSIS OF LOW BACK PAIN

Low back pain is one of the easiest conditions to treat with Prolotherapy. Ninety-five percent of low back pain is located in a 6-by-4 inch area, the weakest link in the vertebral-pelvis complex. At the end of the spine, four structures connect in a very small space which happens to be the 6-by-4 inch area. The fifth lumbar vertebrae connects with the base of the sacrum. This is held together by the lumbosacral ligaments. The sacrum is connected on its sides to the ilium and iliac crest. This is held together by the sacroiliac ligaments. The lumbar vertebrae is held to the iliac crest and ilium by the iliolumbar ligaments. This is typically the area treated with Prolotherapy for chronic low back pain. **(Figure 7-1)**

The diagnosis of ligament laxity in the lower back can be made relatively easily. Typical referral pain patterns are elicited as previously described in Figures 2-2. The sacroiliac ligaments refer pain down the posterior thigh and the lateral foot.[5,6] The sacrotuberous and sacrospinous ligaments refer pain to the heel. The iliolumbar ligament refers pain into the groin or vagina. Iliolumbar ligament sprain should be considered for any unexplained vaginal, testicular, or groin pain.

The first step in determining ligament laxity or instability is by physical examination.[7] The examination involves maneuvering the patient into various stretched positions. If weak ligaments exist, the stressor maneuver will cause pain. Do this simple test at home: Lie flat on your back and lift your legs together as straight and as high as you can, then lower your legs. If it is more painful to lower your legs than to raise them, laxity in the lumbosacral ligaments is likely. The next step is palpating various ligaments with the thumb to elicit tenderness. A positive "jump sign" indicates ligament laxity. *(Refer to Figure 3-5.)*

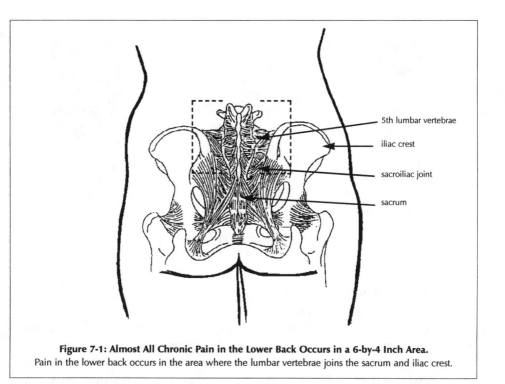

5th lumbar vertebrae

iliac crest

sacroiliac joint

sacrum

Figure 7-1: Almost All Chronic Pain in the Lower Back Occurs in a 6-by-4 Inch Area.
Pain in the lower back occurs in the area where the lumbar vertebrae joins the sacrum and iliac crest.

TREATMENT OF LOW BACK PAIN

The most common cause of unresolved chronic low back pain is injury to the sacroiliac ligaments which typically occurs from bending over and twisting with the knees in a locked, extended position. This maneuver stretches the sacroiliac ligaments, placing them in a vulnerable position.

How effective is Prolotherapy in relieving chronic low back pain? In one of his original papers, George S. Hackett, M.D., noted 82 percent of people treated for posterior sacroiliac ligament relaxation considered themselves cured and remained so 12 years later.[8]

HERNIATED AND DEGENERATED DISC

A herniated disc is a common diagnosis given to patients by their doctors. A person with a degenerated, bulging, or herniated disc must realize that this may be a coincidental finding and unrelated to the actual pain a person is experiencing. A degenerated disc is one that is losing water and flattening. This is a usual phenomenon that occurs with age. It is also normal for a disc to bulge with bending. A herniated disc occurs when the annulus fibrosus no longer holds the gelatinous solution in the disc. The result is a weakened disc. The annulus fibrosus is basically a ring of ligament tissue. What is the best treatment to strengthen ligament tissue? That's right...Prolotherapy.

Why did the disc degenerate in the first place? Degeneration of a disc begins as

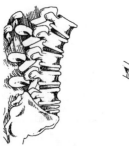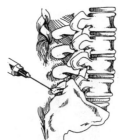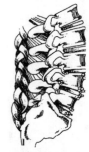

Before Prolotherapy
Weak ligaments cause the vertebrae
to shift putting more pressure on the
disc, making disc herniation more
likely.

During Prolotherapy

After Prolotherapy
The ligaments that support the back
are strong and move the vertebrae
into proper alignment, relieving the
pressure on the discs.

Figure 7-2: Prolotherapy of the Lower Back
Prolotherapy stimulates the growth of soft tissue, such as ligaments and tendons, relieving chronic back pain.

soon as the lumbar ligaments become loose. Once they loosen and weaken, the vertebral segments move excessively and cause pain. The body attempts to correct this by tensing the back muscles. Visits to a chiropractor or medical physician typically begin at this time. The hypermobile vertebral segments add strain to the vertebral discs. Eventually these discs cannot sustain the added pressure and begin to flatten and/or herniate. **(Figure 7-2)** The lumbar ligaments then work harder because the discs no longer cushion the back. A dismal, downward path of pain is the end result.

Prolotherapy is the treatment of choice to strengthen the lumbar vertebral ligaments and prevent the progressive degeneration that occurs with age to the intervertebral discs. Prolotherapy will cause ligament and tendon growth regardless of age. My Prolotherapy patients range from four years of age to 94 years of age. Children and adolescents usually require only one Prolotherapy treatment to resolve a ligament or tendon injury. The young body is already primed to grow new tissue, making Prolotherapy treatments extremely effective.

Adults and the elderly may require more treatments because they are not in the growth mode of life. An adult being treated for chronic pain will receive an average of four sessions of Prolotherapy per area. Those with excellent immune systems will grow more ligament and tendon tissue per session and will therefore require fewer sessions. Those with poor immune systems, especially smokers, require more than the average four sessions. The Prolotherapy treatments are generally given every six weeks to allow the treated area ample time to grow strong ligaments and tendons.

A patient with chronic low back pain is typically treated with Prolotherapy injections into the insertions of the lumbosacral, iliolumbar, and sacroiliac ligaments. The initial assessment may reveal that the chronic low back pain and referred leg pain may be caused by a referred pain from other areas such as the pubic symphysis, hip joint, ischial tuberosity, and sacrospinous and sacrotuberous ligaments. Therefore these areas are also examined.

Off-centered low back pain is often caused by a posterior hip sprain or osteoarthritis of the hip. The hip joint often refers pain to the groin and down the leg to the big toe. Prolotherapy is very effective in this area, often alleviating the necessity for hip replacement surgery.

THE ROLE OF SURGERY

Except in a life-threatening situation or impending neurologic injury, surgery should always be a last resort and done only after all conservative treatments have been exhausted. Pain is not a life-threatening situation. It can be very anxiety-provoking, life-demeaning, and aggravating. Pain should not be an automatic indication that surgery is necessary. Conservative treatments such as vitamins, herbs, massage, physical therapy, chiropractic/osteopathic care, medications, and, of course, Prolotherapy should precede any surgical intervention. Conservative care for back pain is complete only after treatment with Prolotherapy.

It is not uncommon for patients to tell me that surgery has been recommended to resolve their painful back condition. Reasons for surgery may be herniated discs, compressed nerves, spinal stenosis, severe arthritis, and intractable pain. Such conditions may have nothing to do with the problem causing the pain. As previously discussed, abnormalities noted on an MRI scan such as a pinched nerve or herniated disc rarely are the reason I find for someone's chronic back pain. I find that ligament weakness is the number one reason for chronic low back pain, and this diagnosis is not made by an X-ray. It must be made by taking a thorough history and poking the loose ligaments and looking for a positive "jump sign."

Trying conservative treatments before undergoing surgery is only common sense. Surgery is fraught with many potential risks, one being the required anesthesia. General anesthesia greatly stresses the body and complications may occur while under, including kidney and liver failure or a heart attack. A significant percentage of anesthesia-related deaths result from the aspiration (swallowing) of food particles, foreign bodies like dentures, blood, gastric acid, oropharyngeal secretions, or bile during induction of general anesthesia.[9] Other possible complications include damage to the mouth, throat, vocal cords, or lungs from the insertion of the anesthesia tube. If you have ever seen anyone after anesthesia, you know it's no Sunday picnic!

In more than 95 percent of my patients, I find that the true diagnosis causing the pain is different than the diagnosis the patients had been previously given. Rarely will a physician describe a ligament or tendon injury as a cause of chronic pain. Remember, ligaments and tendons often do not appear on X-rays. The diagnosis of ligament or tendon weakness cannot be made by a blood test, electrical test, or X-ray. It must be made using a listening ear and a strong thumb.

Even back in early 1981 as new and more effective methods of conservative treatments were being used (including Prolotherapy), the need for surgery was decreasing. Bernard E. Finneson, M.D., pointed out in a survey of surgical cases that "80% should not... have been brought to surgery." It is quite possible that with the widespread use of Prolotherapy this percentage would be even higher.[10]

In more than 95 percent of pain cases, surgery can be avoided by utilizing Prolotherapy. Dr. Hemwall, having treated more than 10,000 pain patients, resorted

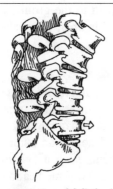

Figure 7-3A: Spondylolisthesis or Subluxation of the Lower Back
Weakened ligaments cause vertebrae to slip which could lead to pinching of a nerve.

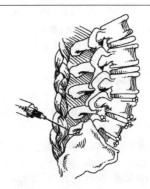

Figure 7-3B: After Prolotherapy All the Vertebrae Have Proper Alignment
Proper alignment of vertebrae relieves nerve pinching.

to surgery for resolving a chronic pain complaint in only one percent of the patients. My experience has been similar. In the event that surgery is necessary, the previous Prolotherapy treatment will not hinder the subsequent surgical procedure. Prolotherapy causes normal ligament and tendon tissue to form. The surgeon will observe an area treated with Prolotherapy containing strengthened ligament and tendon tissue.

PINCHED OR COMPRESSED NERVES

Another cause of back pain, although rare, may be a pinched or compressed nerve. A wonderful conservative treatment for this condition is chiropractic/osteopathic manipulation. These therapies have a high success rate for acutely compressed nerve cases because bony malalignment (subluxation) of the vertebrae is often the reason the nerve is pinched.

Why did the vertebral bones slip out of alignment? The answer is ligament laxity which causes the vertebrae to slip out of place and pinch the nerve. Nerve blocks utilizing a 70.0 percent Sarapin and 0.6 percent Lidocaine solution are often given, in addition to Prolotherapy, for this condition. This solution will relax the nerve, providing pain relief, while Prolotherapy grows ligament tissue. Upon nerve relaxation, the vertebrae will realign and the nerve compression will cease. A series of Prolotherapy treatments along with nerve blocks will usually resolve the pain. **(Figure 7-3)**

I ask people considering surgery to exhaust all conservative treatments, including Prolotherapy, before succumbing to surgical intervention. Surgery removes tissue. Prolotherapy repairs tissue. The discs, the bones, and the joints are there for a reason. Surgical procedures removing tissue in an attempt to alleviate lower back pain will almost always leave a long-term detrimental effect on the body. Surgery ultimately makes the body weaker by removing tissue, whereas Prolotherapy makes the body stronger by growing tissue.

PROLOTHERAPY VERSUS SURGERY: A STUDY

In 1964, John R. Merriman, M.D., compared Prolotherapy versus operative fusion in the treatment of instability of the spine and pelvis and wrote, "The purpose of this article is to evaluate the merit of two methods of treating instability of the spine and pelvis, with which I have been concerned during 40 years as a general and industrial surgeon.... The success of either method depends on regeneration of bone cells to provide joint stabilization, elimination of pain and resumption of activity ... Ligament and tendon relaxation occurs when the fibro-osseous attachments to bone do not regain their normal tensile strength after sprain and lacerations, and when the attachments are weakened by decalcification from disease, menopause and aging."[11]

The figure below describes Dr. Merriman's results:[12]

Areas Effected	Response to Prolotherapy (Physiologic Treatment)	Response to Fusion Operation (Mechanical Treatment)
New Bone	Prompt	Retarded
Ligaments	Strengthened	Excised (Removed)
Tendons	Strengthened	Incised (Cut)
Spinous Process	Strengthened	Sacrificed
Joint Motion	Preserved	Abolished
Pain	Eliminated	May Continue
Loss of Time	Negligible	Considerable
Results	80-90 Percent Cures	Variable

Dr. Merriman summarized that conservative physiologic treatment by Prolotherapy after a confirmed diagnosis of ligamental and tendinous relaxation was successful in 80 to 90 percent of more than 15,000 patients treated.

TYPES OF BACK SURGERY

1. Laminectomy. The most common back surgery is a laminectomy. This surgical procedure involves removing some of the bone, called lamina, from the supporting structure of the back. Its removal creates stress on other areas of the lumbar spine.

Because some of the lamina are removed, the discs, ligaments, and muscles have to do more work. As a result, the vertebral discs degenerate. The vertebral segments then move closer together and eventually become hypermobile. Back muscles tense to stabilize the segment. When they cannot stabilize the segments, the vertebral ligaments are then forced to do this alone. They eventually become lax and subsequently cause pain. This is probably why back pain so commonly occurs several years after this operation. If the muscles and ligaments cannot stabilize the joints in the lower back, the vertebrae loosen and eventually rub together and crack, causing excessive bone growth in order to stabilize the joint. The stabilization results in spondylosis, or arthritis of the lumbar spine. Often the person then succumbs to another operation for the arthritis that formed as a result of the first operation. Unfortunately for the patient, the second operation isn't a panacea of pain relief

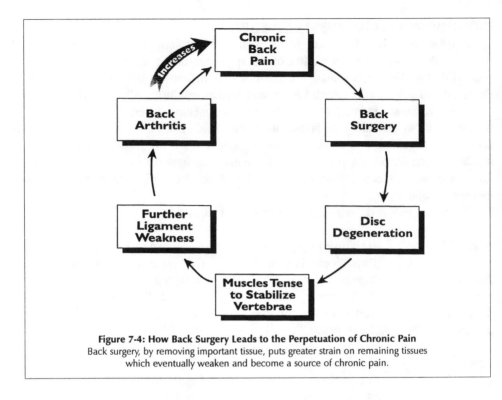

Figure 7-4: How Back Surgery Leads to the Perpetuation of Chronic Pain
Back surgery, by removing important tissue, puts greater strain on remaining tissues
which eventually weaken and become a source of chronic pain.

either. A simpler approach is Prolotherapy to correct the underlying ligament laxity which was causing the pain in the first place. This sequence of events is also applicable to other areas of the body. **(Figure 7-4)**

2. Discectomy. Discectomy, another common back surgery, follows the same degenerative sequence as a laminectomy. Once the disc material is surgically removed, stress is added to the segments above and below the removed disc segment. These segments may eventually degenerate and become a cause of chronic pain. In a study by John Maynard, M.D., 10 percent of people after disc operation reherniated the same disc at a later date. Four years after surgery, 38 percent of the patients still had persistent pain in the back and 23 percent had persistent pain in the lower limbs.[13]

3. Lumbar spinal fusion. Lumbar spinal fusion operations fuse together several segments of the vertebrae. Such an operation is commonly performed for spondylolisthesis, a condition where one vertebral segment slips forward on another. **(Figure 7-3)** This causes back pain, especially when bending. By definition, spinal fusion causes permanent bonding or fusing of several vertebral segments. Mobility is decreased, causing increased stress on the areas above and below the fused segment. Over time, this stress may create weakened ligaments. The weakened ligaments lead to a degenerated disc which eventually leads to a degenerated spine resulting in a painfully stiff back.

Prolotherapy is a much safer and effective alternative to a laminectomy, a discectomy, or a lumbar spinal fusion. Prolotherapy initiates the repair process of the

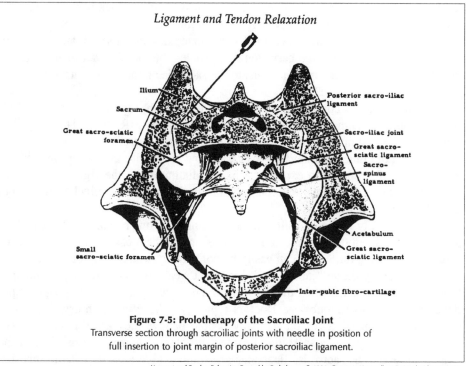

Ligament and Tendon Relaxation

Figure 7-5: Prolotherapy of the Sacroiliac Joint
Transverse section through sacroiliac joints with needle in position of
full insertion to joint margin of posterior sacroiliac ligament.

loose ligaments in spondylolisthesis and degenerated and herniated discs. For these reasons, Prolotherapy should be performed before a patient considers a surgical procedure to alleviate pain.

In her article, published in the *Journal of the American Medical Association* in 1992, "Patient Outcomes After Lumbar Spinal Fusions," Judith A. Turner, Ph.D., noted that there has never been a randomized or double-blind study comparing lumbar spinal fusion with any other technique. In some cases, only 16 percent of the people experienced satisfactory results after the operation. On average, 14 percent of the people experience incomplete healing of the surgical site. The most frequent symptom persisting after the operation is low back pain, which is often the reason for the operation in the first place. Turner concluded her article by saying that the wide variability in reported success rates is bothersome and should be carefully considered by patients and their physicians when contemplating this procedure.[14]

PROLOTHERAPY AFTER BACK SURGERY

Many people only become aware of Prolotherapy after they have undergone a surgical procedure for back pain. Although the pain may not be as severe as it was before the surgery, most people continue to experience significant back pain after surgery. Why? The back surgery involved removing supporting structure(s) such as a lamina, facet, or disc thus weakening surrounding segments.

Prolotherapy injections to the weakened segments in the lumbar vertebrae often result in definitive pain relief in post-surgery pain syndromes. Back pain is commonly due to several factors and surgery may have eliminated only one. It is possible, for example, to have back pain from a lumbar herniated disc and a sacroiliac joint problem. Surgery may address the herniated disc problem but not the sacroiliac problem. In this example, Prolotherapy injections to the sacroiliac joint would cure the chronic pain problem. **(Figure 7-5)**

Unfortunately it is common for a person to have lumbar spine surgery for a "sciatica" complaint diagnosed from an "abnormality" on an MRI scan. The "sciatica" complaint was a simple ligament problem in the sacroiliac joint and the MRI scan finding was not clinically relevant—it had nothing to do with the pain problem. For the majority of people who experience pain radiating down the leg, even in cases where numbness is present, the cause of the problem is not a pinched nerve but sacroiliac ligament weakness.

Ligament laxity in the sacroiliac joint is the number one reason for "sciatica" or pain radiating down the side of the leg, and is one of the most common reasons for chronic low back pain.[15] This can easily be confirmed by stretching these ligaments and producing a positive "jump sign." Ligament weakness can cause leg numbness. Most people sense pain when they have ligament weakness, but some people experience a sensation of numbness. Doctors typically believe nerve injury is the only reason for numbness, a reason so many people believe they have a sciatic nerve problem. In reality it is a sacroiliac ligament problem. The referral patterns of the sciatic nerve and the sacroiliac ligaments are similar. (*See Figures 2-2.*) In this scenario, it is unfortunate that thousands of dollars were spent on surgery and post-operative care. Had Prolotherapy treatments been performed on the pain-producing structure, this could have been avoided.

DIAGNOSIS OF ARACHNOIDITIS

Arachnoiditis is typically diagnosed in someone who has undergone back surgery and still suffers severe back pain that radiates down the legs and often to the feet. The pain has a persistent burning, stinging, or aching quality.[16] The diagnosis is occasionally made when similar symptoms are felt in the neck, arms, or the mid back with radiation into the chest. This pain is typically unresponsive to pain medications and muscle relaxants.

The term arachnoiditis signifies an inflammation of the arachnoid membrane which covers the spinal cord. The diagnosis of arachnoiditis is generally inaccurate because no signs of inflammation such as redness, fever, or an elevated sed rate (blood test that identifies inflammation) are seen in these patients. All that is seen is scar tissue on the MRI.

Arachnoiditis is another condition that is typically diagnosed by the large metal box with a magnet in it. For the patient who succumbed to surgery, only to be left with continued or worsened leg pains, repeated MRI and CAT scans are done. Eventually one of these scans will show some scar tissue. The physician will then inform the patient that the mysterious cause of the pain has been found, "You have arachnoiditis. Scar tissue is pinching the nerves."

It is common for someone with severe burning pains in the legs to receive a diagnostic study such as an MRI or CAT scan of the lower back. These tests are performed because they are supposed to reveal the source of the problem to the physician. The problem with this logic is that the MRI or CAT scan is designed to reveal density and configuration of structures, not diagnose conditions. Physicians are supposed to diagnose but unfortunately for many people with chronic pain, physicians have left the diagnosing to a large metal box with a magnet in it.

The patient in the above scenario is at first ecstatic because "the cause" of the pain has been found. The patient's jubilation is short-lived when the physician tells the patient that arachnoiditis is not curable, but the pain can be "controlled." Imagine having surgery for back and leg pain and coming out of the surgery with the same back and leg pain. The doctor then says the pain is due to scar tissue pinching on the nerves. How did the scar tissue get there? The answer is from the surgery of course.

The problem with this diagnosis is that the scar tissue was not present before the surgery, but the back and leg pains were. So what explains the back and leg pain that occurred before surgery? Answer that one and you will have the answer to why the person suffers from back and leg pain after surgery.

A more logical conclusion is that the surgery did not address the cause of the back and leg pain. Furthermore, the scar tissue seen on X-ray most likely has nothing to do with the current pain complaints of the patient. The number one cause of low back pain radiating into the legs is sacroiliac ligament laxity. Shooting pain down the leg is commonly due to ligament weakness in the lower back, including the sacroiliac, iliolumbar, sacrospinous, sacrotuberous, and hip joint ligaments. (*See Figures 2-2.*)

The person in the above scenario needed a Prolotherapist to relieve the pain, not a surgeon. Anyone carrying the diagnosis of arachnoiditis needs the immediate attention of a Prolotherapist before succumbing to epidural steroid injections, more surgeries, spinal cord stimulator implantation, or other invasive treatments which are only marginally helpful.[17,18]

Arachnoiditis has been described as occurring after invasive treatments in and around the spinal column such as neck or back surgery, cortisone injections, spinal anesthetics, or myelography (a technique whereby dye is injected around the spinal cord to visualize the nerves).[19] The question is what percentage of people will develop a scar as evidenced on X-ray after back surgery? If you said 100 percent, you are correct. Each time a person undergoes surgery, a scar will develop. It is that simple.

Many people with the diagnosis of arachnoiditis have a repeat surgery to remove the scar tissue that is pinching on the nerves. Unfortunately, the results after a second surgery are dismal when it comes to permanent pain relief.

RESEARCH STUDY

A study consisting of 36 patients with arachnoiditis noted that each patient averaged three previous myelograms and three back surgeries.[20] They endured three pokes in the back for the myelogram and three knife treatments. Don't you think your X-ray would show scar tissue after all of that?! In this study, 88 percent of the patients were diagnosed with arachnoiditis by X-ray and the other 12 percent by

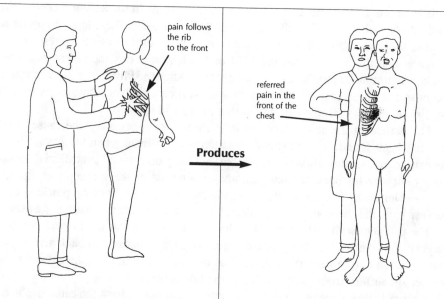

Produces

**Figure 7-6A: Physician Reproduces Pain
at the Rib-Vertebrae Junction**
Weakness at the rib-vertebrae (costovertebral) junction
ligaments are a common source of mid-back pain.

**Figure 7-6B: Referral Pain Pattern
of the Rib-Sternal Junction**
Rib-vertebrae (costovertebral) ligament weakness
can cause pain to occur in the chest.

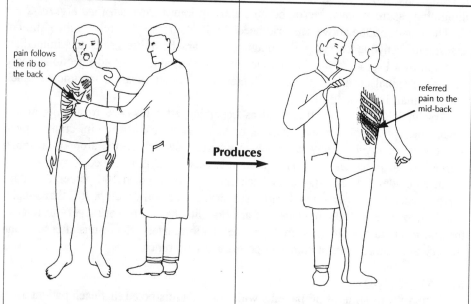

Produces

**Figure 7-6C: Physician Reproduces Pain
at the Rib-Sternal Junction**
Weakness at the rib-sternal (costochondral
or sternocostal) junction ligaments is
a common source of chest pain.

**Figure 7-6D: Referral Pain Pattern
of the Rib-Vertebrae Junction**
Rib-sternal (costochondral or sternocostal)
ligament weakness can cause pain to occur
in the side or mid-back region.

surgery. Do you see a problem? What about a patient history? What about the thumb? A few pokes on the sacroiliac joint eliciting a positive "jump sign" and the cause of the pain would have been accurately identified.

Often people with the diagnosis of "arachnoiditis" experience significant difficulties in walking or holding down a job. The most startling result observed from the study was that the average life span was shortened by 12 years. Anyone who has had back surgery with recurrent pain should be evaluated for another cause of the pain besides arachnoiditis. Since scar tissue occurs 100 percent of the time after surgery, an MRI showing scar tissue should not be used to make a diagnosis. People who carry this diagnosis usually have the history of repeated tests and invasive procedures with the end result being a life expectancy shortened by 12 years.

Prolotherapy to the weakened structures such as the sacroiliac ligaments causing the pain will cure the condition and alleviate the pain. Once the weakened structure in the back becomes strong, the pain stops. Once the pain stops, the CAT and MRI scans and subsequent surgeries also stop. Consequently, many people with arachnoiditis are choosing to Prolo their pain away.

MID-UPPER BACK PAIN

James Cade, M.D., described the following case to me: "W.M., a 34-year-old with severe mid-upper back pain between the shoulder blades, found no relief despite chronic use of Vicodin pain pills. The MRI, regular X-ray, and bone scan of W.M.'s thoracic spine showed no abnormalities. W.M. was offered surgery, costing $28,000, with little hope of success. I palpated the costovertebral ligaments and reproduced his pain. He agreed to the Prolotherapy injections and was on the way to healing his chronic pain."

This case illustrates many important points concerning routine chronic pain management. It is common for people to be offered surgery because nothing else has helped. Surgery should never be considered as routine as slicing a ham sandwich. Surgery involves someone cutting, slicing, grinding, tearing, and pulling out your body parts while you're asleep. It is my contention that if people were shown a video of the surgery prior to the operation, few would consent. No one should have surgery "just to try it." Surgery should only be performed for chronic pain management in the most extreme circumstances and only if all other conservative treatments have not been successful.

Most of the body's ligaments are not revealed on X-ray. The diagnosis of ligament injury is made by history and physical examination, not by X-ray. Dr. Cade was familiar with ligament injuries and their referral patterns and prevented W.M. from an unnecessary operation that in all likelihood would not have solved the problem. W.M. had ligament weakness at the rib-vertebrae junction, allowing his ribs to move too much which further stretched his costovertebral ligaments leading to more pain. Costovertebral ligament laxity often refers pain from the mid-upper back to the chest. **(Figures 7-6)** This is one of the causes for chronic chest discomfort.

Costovertebral ligament injuries are very slow to heal, or heal incompletely, because they are constantly under stress from the movement of the rib cage during

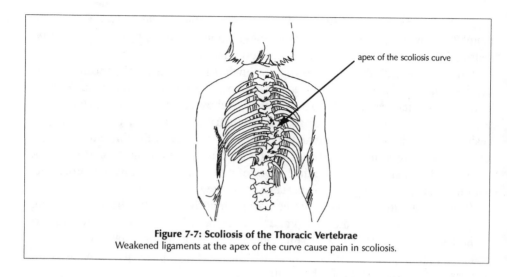

Figure 7-7: Scoliosis of the Thoracic Vertebrae
Weakened ligaments at the apex of the curve cause pain in scoliosis.

breathing. The costovertebral junctions are prone to being injured any time the rib cage is jarred. This may occur from being hit in the chest, after receiving CPR, or from the effects of heart or thoracic surgery. During these types of surgeries the sternum is opened and the ribs are spread apart, commonly causing injury to the costovertebral junctions. In my opinion, chronic chest or upper-back discomfort after heart or lung surgery is almost always due to injury to the ligament support at the rib attachments in the thoracic spine or on the sternum. Prolotherapy is extremely effective at eliminating post-bypass chest or upper-back discomfort.

Prolotherapy, as in the case illustrated, is extremely effective at stabilizing vertebral segments and vertebral-rib segments. Costovertebral ligament laxity is a common cause of chronic mid-upper back or chest pain. This is why many people are choosing to Prolo their chronic mid-upper back and chest pain away.

PAIN FROM SCOLIOSIS

Scoliosis is a lateral curvature of the spine of 11 degrees or more. An estimated 500,000 adults in the United States have scoliosis.[21] Scoliosis is usually discovered during adolescence and is called idiopathic scoliosis, a fancy term meaning the doctor has no idea what caused the scoliosis.

In common language, scoliosis means that the spine is crooked. The spine is held together by the same thing that holds all the bones together, ligaments. The patient often experiences pain at the site where the spine curves. At the apex of this curve, the ligaments are being stretched with the scoliosis, and localized ligament weakness is one of the etiological bases for it.

Traditional treatments for scoliosis, especially during adolescence, include observation, bracing, and surgery.[22,23,24] Observation of a crooked spine does not sound very helpful, bracing has been shown to decrease the progression of mild scoliosis, and surgery involves placing big rods in the back to stabilize the spine. Surgery is generally utilized for severe scoliosis when bracing has failed to stop the progression.

Again, every disease has a cause. Since scoliosis involves the spine moving in the wrong direction, treatment should be aimed at why this is occurring and correcting the problem. Ligament laxity is probably the main plausible explanation for the development of scoliosis and its pain. Prolotherapy treatments to strengthen the weakened ligaments can have potentially stabilizing and curative effects in scoliosis. If the scoliosis is progressing quickly, then bracing would be necessary in addition to Prolotherapy.

Scoliosis pain has common patterns depending on where the scoliosis is located.[25] These pain patterns are easily reproduced by palpating the ligaments over the scoliotic segments of the spine. A positive "jump sign" will be elicited ensuring the diagnosis. The most common reason for pain with scoliosis is ligament weakness at the apex of the scoliosis curve. **(Figure 7-7)** Prolotherapy treatments over the entire scoliotic segment is effective at eliminating the pain of scoliosis. It has the added benefit of causing the ligaments to strengthen which will help stabilize the segment. For these reasons, Prolotherapy should be a part of comprehensive scoliosis management.

SUMMARY

In summary, the treatment that should be utilized in resistant cases of back pain is Prolotherapy. Prolotherapy eliminates chronic back pain in conditions such as degenerated discs, herniated discs, spondylolisthesis, post-surgery pain syndromes, arachnoiditis, and scoliosis. The most common cause of chronic low back pain and "sciatica" is laxity of the sacroiliac ligaments. Prolotherapy should be tried before any surgical procedure is performed for chronic back pain. Prolotherapy is an extremely effective treatment for chronic low back pain because it permanently strengthens the structures that are causing the pain. It is for this reason that many people are choosing to Prolo their chronic back pain away.

CHAPTER 8

Prolo Your Headache, Neck, TMJ, Ear, and Mouth Pain Away

Most chronic pain commonly occurs in either the neck region or the lower back. This is most likely due in part to the stresses of life which seem to accumulate in these two areas. Unfortunately for many people who have chronic neck pain, the diagnosis of muscle tension pain is given. Doctors "pooh-pooh" the complaint and tell the person that the condition is all stress-related. This may be partly true, but does nothing to help cure the problem.

As with pain in all other body parts, neck, headache, and facial pain are almost always caused by weakness in a soft tissue structure. Ligament weakness in the neck accounts for the majority of chronic headaches, neck, ear, and mouth pain. Because Prolotherapy stimulates the growth of the weakened ligament causing the pain, many people obtain permanent pain relief with this treatment. No matter if it's migraine, cluster, or tension headaches, Prolotherapy can help decrease or even eliminate the pain associated with these conditions.

HEADACHE PAIN
Migraines

I could see that another Saturday night was about to be ruined when a migraine headache began taking away my wife's cheery disposition. She claims her migraine headaches started the day we were married. I, of course, know this was purely coincidental, as Marion has the most giving and wonderful husband.

Migraine headaches tend to take over a family. If one member is "out" with a migraine headache another member is helping them cope. Anyone who has experienced a migraine headache or has seen a loved one suffer through a migraine attack knows it is a most unpleasant experience.

Typical medical management of migraine headaches involves the avoidance of various foods like chocolate, tyramine-containing cheese, and alcoholic beverages.[1] Various medications are used in an attempt to abort the migraine once it has started. Prophylactic medications, such as Propranolol, are used in an attempt to prevent the dreaded migraine. Unfortunately, a migraine headache is not due to a Propranolol deficiency. Neither is it an aspirin, Motrin, Tylenol, Imitrex, or Elavil deficiency. Migraine headaches have a cause and that cause can be determined by a careful examination. The cause of migraine headaches can nearly always be found by a good listening ear and a strong thumb.

Causes of Migraines

If the migraine headaches occur at a particular part of a woman's menstrual cycle, a hormonal abnormality is likely involved. The hormonal abnormality is usually due to a low progesterone level during the second half of the menstrual cycle. Giving natural progesterone during this part of the menstrual cycle will often relieve the problem. (*Refer to Appendix C, Natural Medicine Resources, for organizations that can give you the names of Natural Medicine Clinics familiar with Natural Hormone Replacement Therapy.*)

If the migraine headaches occur when eating particular foods, during particular times of the year, or when exposed to certain scents, an allergic component to the migraines should be investigated. Migraine headaches are a common symptom of food allergies. Eliminating the suspect food from the diet will likely solve the migraine problem. In my clinic, I use Metabolic Typing to test the pH of the blood, urine, and saliva of patients experiencing migraine headaches. Balancing a patient's pH is generally very helpful in eliminating migraine headaches. (*Refer to Appendix A, Nutrition and Chronic Pain, to learn more about Metabolic Typing and Balancing Body Chemistry.*)

Treatments of Migraines

Current traditional drugs for migraine headaches, such as Ergotamine, Fiorinal, Codeine, and the other medications, provide only temporary relief. The patient dependent on these drugs for headache relief lives in fear of the next migraine attack. Patients describe their migraine headaches as similar to having one half of their head hit repeatedly with a baseball bat.

On the particular Saturday night described above, my wife finally agreed to let me administer Prolotherapy injections to the back of her head and neck. I had been using Prolotherapy in my practice for about a year at the time. Our living room couch was transformed into an examining table. In 10 minutes, my wife had completed her first Prolotherapy session. Her migraine headache immediately vanished. Two additional treatments were necessary to make the formerly weekly migraine headaches a rarity.

Prolotherapy is the best curative treatment for migraine headaches. Often the migraine sufferer will say that neck pain or tightness is associated with the migraine and will signal the start of the headache. This is a sign that the source of the migraine is in the neck. I have personally treated hundreds of patients with migraine headaches. Only one did not have a positive response to Prolotherapy. The success rate of Prolotherapy in the total elimination of migraine headaches is at least 90 percent. I'm sure such a high percentage will seem unrealistic to some people, but this claim is dependent upon an accurate diagnosis. If the primary cause of the migraine headache stems from ligament or tendon injury in the neck, a high success rate with Prolotherapy is expected.

Sometimes a person has other factors, in addition to ligament weakness in the neck, associated with initiating the migraines, including food sensitivities, hormone deficiencies, and yeast infections. In these instances, Prolotherapy must be combined with Natural Medicine techniques, such as elimination of allergic foods from the diet, natural hormone supplementation, or yeast infection treatment to obtain completely curative results.

People who have suffered for years can still find relief with Prolotherapy. Prolotherapy has helped thousands of people with tension, migraine, cluster, and other nagging headaches.

"I had cluster migraine headaches off and on for about 16 years," said Kendall Gill, Guard for the New Jersey Nets basketball team. "The headaches would last for one to two months. It did not matter how many pain pills or pain shots I took. They would only return with a vengeance. They would hamper my daily activities to the point where all I could do was stand still and hope the pain would go away." After receiving one Prolotherapy treatment by Gustav A. Hemwall, M.D., the world's most experienced Prolotherapist, Kendall Gill was headache-free for two years.

After a flare-up of his headache pain, Kendall Gill knew where to turn, and it was not to the local pharmacist. He learned that headaches are not due to a pain pill deficiency. Headaches, even cluster and migraine headaches, have a definitive cause. The most common cause of headache pain is ligament laxity in the neck. The best treatment option for long-term curative results is Prolotherapy because it addresses the underlying cause of the problem, ligament weakness.

Kendall Gill had one more Prolotherapy session on his neck and head region and has been headache-free since. "I wish I had known about it [Prolotherapy] 16 years ago," he says. "I recommend it for anyone suffering with headaches."

BARRÉ-LIEOU SYNDROME (HEADACHE WITH CHRONIC SINUSITIS/ALLERGIES)

Early in his Prolotherapy practice, Dr. Hemwall noted some interesting phenomena occurring after Prolotherapy injections. His patients' neck pain was relieved with Prolotherapy and to his surprise their dizziness, headaches, nausea, blurred vision, and tinnitus (ringing in the ears) were also alleviated. A few patients even had improvements in their vision after receiving Prolotherapy injections to their neck. People who suffer from chronic sinus congestion may find immediate relief from Prolotherapy treatment in the neck. Other serendipitous findings included improvement in paresthesias (pin pricking sensations in the arms), generalized weakness, and ear, face, and tongue pain. The reason for this was puzzling until Dr. Hemwall learned about Barré-Lieou Syndrome.[2]

In 1925, Jean Alexandre Barré, M.D., a French Neurologist, and in 1928, Yong-Choen Lieou, a Chinese physician, each independently described a syndrome with a variety of symptoms thought to be due to a dysfunction in the posterior cervical sympathetic nervous system. The posterior cervical sympathetic syndrome became known as the Barré-Lieou Syndrome. The posterior cervical sympathetic nervous system is a group of nerves located near the vertebrae in the neck.

Symptoms that characterize the Barré-Lieou Syndrome are listed below.[3,4]

- Headache
- Vertigo
- Hoarseness
- Sinus Congestion
- Facial pain
- Tinnitus
- Neck pain
- Chest pain
- Ear pain
- Loss of voice
- Severe fatigue
- Sense of eyeball being pulled out

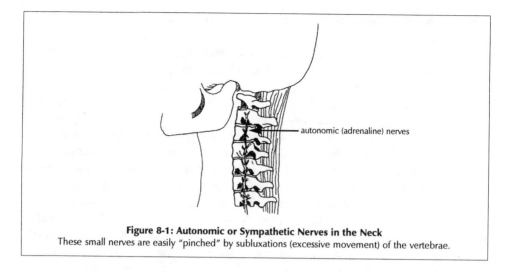

Figure 8-1: Autonomic or Sympathetic Nerves in the Neck
These small nerves are easily "pinched" by subluxations (excessive movement) of the vertebrae.

Other symptoms may include dysesthesias of the hands and forearms (painful pins and needles sensation), corneal sensitivity, dental pain, lacrimation (tearing of the eyes), blurred vision, facial numbness, shoulder pain, swelling of one side of the face, nausea, vomiting, and localized cyanosis of the face (bluish color).

A reasonable question to ask is how can one disorder cause all of these problems? The answer lies in understanding the function of the sympathetic nervous system which is part of the autonomic nervous system. The autonomic nervous system operates automatically. That is why it is called the autonomic nervous system. It keeps your heart pumping, your blood flowing through your blood vessels, your lungs breathing, and a myriad of other activities that occur in your body all the time, every day of your life. The sympathetic nervous system is part of the autonomic nervous system. It is activated when the body is "on alert." For instance, if you are being robbed your body shifts into "fight mode." Your heart rate, blood pressure, and breathing rate dramatically increase. The blood vessels shift blood away from the intestines into the muscles, enabling you to run or fight the offender.

The posterior cervical sympathetic system signals the sympathetic part of the autonomic nervous system that controls the head, neck, and face area. In the Barré-Lieou Syndrome, the posterior cervical sympathetic system is underactive because the vertebrae in the neck are pinching the sympathetic nerves. **(Figure 8-1)**

What symptoms are produced in the face, head, and neck when the sympathetic system is not working well in these areas? The primary symptom is a headache, since headaches are caused by dilation of blood vessels, as in Barré-Lieou Syndrome. The main medicines used to abort severe headache pain, as in migraines, are Cafergot, Ergotamine, and Sumatriptin, all of which **vasoconstrict** the blood vessels. These medicines work, but only temporarily. The medicines act on the symptom of the dysfunction, but not the cause. Thus, the benefit is only temporary. Prolotherapy to the vertebrae in the neck is the treatment of choice to permanently eliminate Barré-Lieou Syndrome. This occurs because Prolotherapy causes the vertebrae in the neck to

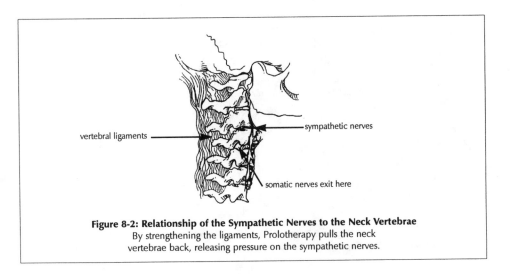

Figure 8-2: Relationship of the Sympathetic Nerves to the Neck Vertebrae
By strengthening the ligaments, Prolotherapy pulls the neck
vertebrae back, releasing pressure on the sympathetic nerves.

move posteriorly (back) and no longer pinch the sympathetic nerves. **(Figure 8-2)**

Another symptom of Barré-Lieou Syndrome is tinnitus (ringing in the ears). A decrease in sympathetic output to the inner ear will cause an accumulation of fluid in the inner ear. When fluid accumulates in the inner ear, as is often the case with an upper respiratory infection, the ear feels full and the body feels off balance. A ringing in the ear can occur, along with vertigo (dizziness). When Prolotherapy is performed on the head and neck, the posterior sympathetic nervous system begins to function correctly. Conditions such as dizziness, tinnitus, and vertigo (Meniere's Disease) can all be eliminated with Prolotherapy if the symptoms are due to Barré-Lieou Syndrome.

If sympathetic output to the sinus area is low, fluid will also accumulate in this area. Often immediately after Prolotherapy injections to the posterior head and neck areas, patients with Barré-Lieou Syndrome, who have had sinus trouble for years, experience clear breathing which they have not had in years. People using decongestants for years for "chronic allergies" and "chronic sinus infections" are often immediately helped by Prolotherapy injections into the head and neck region.

The other symptoms such as blurred vision, severe fatigue, dysesthesias (pins and needles down the arm), low blood pressure, and low heart rate are easily understood by a decrease in the output of the sympathetic system of the head, neck and face areas. Prolotherapy injections to the head and neck region cause the vertebrae to realign which decreases the compression of the nerves. Upon realignment, the Barré-Lieou Syndrome and its symptomatology are abated.

Causes and Diagnosis

Barré-Lieou Syndrome occurs because of ligament weakness in the neck. Signs of ligament weakness in the neck are chronic neck pain, decreased range of motion of the neck, a head forward posture, and difficulty in keeping the head supported on its own during a lecture, "boring lecture syndrome." Look around a classroom

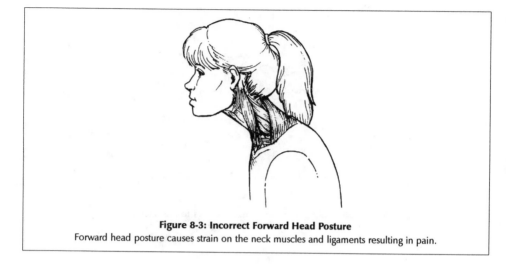

Figure 8-3: Incorrect Forward Head Posture
Forward head posture causes strain on the neck muscles and ligaments resulting in pain.

and notice the people with weak neck ligaments. They are the people with head forward posture supporting their heads with their hands.

Ligament weakness in the neck can occur suddenly, such as after a whiplash injury during a car accident, or more commonly occurring slowly over time.

Daniel Kayfetz, M.D., reported treating 189 patients from March 1956 through May 1961 with Prolotherapy who had whiplash injuries to their necks. Fifty-two percent had associated sympathetic nervous system symptoms as seen in Barré-Lieou Syndrome, 55 percent of the people had symptoms longer than three months, 81 percent had symptoms and injuries in other parts of the body in addition to the neck, and 49 percent had some kind of legal action because of an auto accident they were in (79 percent were involved in auto accidents). By all practical purposes these were not simple cases of neck strain yet Prolotherapy totally eliminated the pain in 60 percent of the patients, and 86 percent of the patients considered the end result to be satisfactory (in other words they had pain relief with the Prolotherapy).[5]

Barré-Lieou Syndrome can also be a late sequela of whiplash injury. C.F. Claussen noted that in Germany in 1992 they had 197,731 cases of whiplash injuries due to traffic accidents. About 80 percent recovered within a few months. However about "…15-20% developed the so-called *late whiplash injury syndrome* with many complaints of the cervico-encephalic syndrome including headache, vertigo, instability, nausea, tinnitus, hearing loss, etc." It is evident that these symptoms are compatible with Barré-Lieou Syndrome and this explains why Prolotherapy is so effective in treating whiplash injury and its sequelae.[6]

Barré-Lieou Syndrome more commonly occurs because most people spend a good portion of their day hunched over while working. Their work may consist of typing on a computer, punching buttons on a cash register, or balancing a check book. All of these activities precipitate the head forward position and put the cervical vertebral ligaments in a stretched position. **(Figure 8-3)** Over time, these ligaments weaken and cause pain. The ligament laxity causes an even more head forward position as the

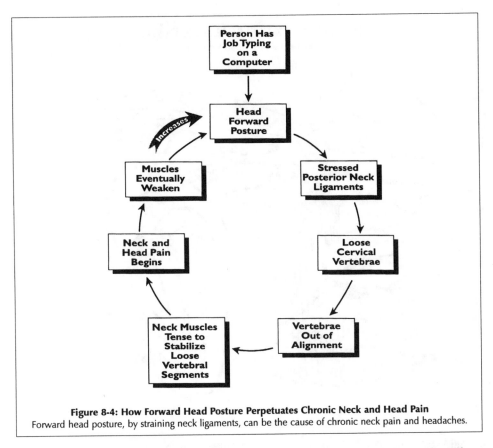

Figure 8-4: How Forward Head Posture Perpetuates Chronic Neck and Head Pain
Forward head posture, by straining neck ligaments, can be the cause of chronic neck pain and headaches.

ligaments can no longer keep the cervical vertebrae in their proper posterior alignment. The paracervical muscles (the neck muscles) tighten to stabilize the joints and head. As the muscles tighten, they create more pain. Eventually the muscles can no longer stabilize the vertebrae and the ligaments are stretched even more. Neck pain increases and the cycle continues to repeat itself. **(Figure 8-4)** Massage therapy, physical therapy, chiropractic/osteopathic manipulation, and pain medicines all help to temporarily relieve the pain. They do not, however, correct the underlying problem of ligament laxity. Prolotherapy addresses the root cause of neck pain, ligament laxity, and is consequently effective at eliminating the problem.

Neck and Headache Treatments

Most people say a headache starts at the base of the neck, moves up the neck, behind the eyes, in the temples, and into the head. Migraine sufferers know that pain on one side in the base of the neck may be the beginning of a migraine headache. This is an important clue that the etiology of the headache is in the neck producing referred pain. George S. Hackett, M.D., the father of Prolotherapy, described the referral patterns of the ligaments of the neck in detail. **(Figure 8-5)** These patterns are important to know because the most common cause for pain radiating from the

HEAD AND NECK REFERRAL PAIN PATTERNS
Ligament and Tendon Relaxation

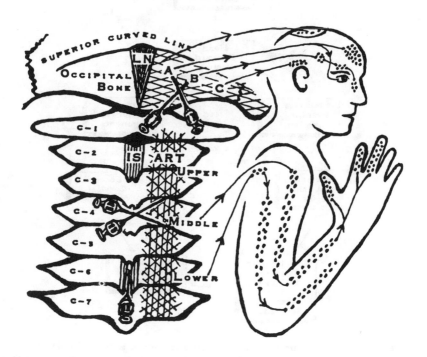

AREA OF WEAKNESS	REFERRAL PATTERN
Occiput Area A	Forehead and Eye
Occiput Area B	Temple, Eyebrow, and Nose
Occiput Area C	Above the Ear
Cervical Vertebrae #1 – #3 (Upper)	Back of Neck and Posterior Scapular Region (Not Shown)
Cervical Vertebrae #4 – #5 (Middle)	Lateral Arm and Forearm Into the Thumb, Index, and Middle Finger
Cervical Vertebrae #6 – #7 (Lower)	Medial Arm and Forearm Into the Lateral Hand, Ring, and Little Finger

Figure 8-5: Hackett Referral Patterns
Head and neck ligament referral pain patterns.

Ligament and Tendon Relaxation Treated by Prolotherapy © 1991, Gustav A. Hemwall, M.D. Used with permission.

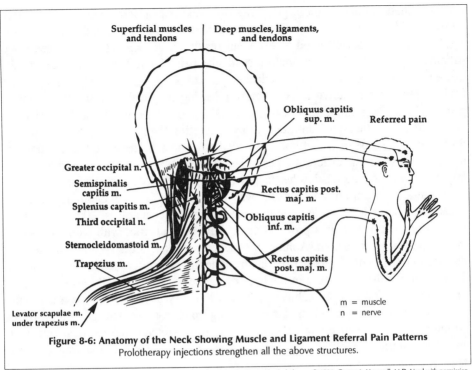

Figure 8-6: Anatomy of the Neck Showing Muscle and Ligament Referral Pain Patterns
Prolotherapy injections strengthen all the above structures.

neck to the arm is not a pinched nerve in the neck, but actually a weak ligament in the neck. The most common reason for a pins and needles sensation or numbness in the arm is not a pinched nerve, but ligament laxity in the neck.

To accurately diagnose the cause of neck or head pain, a listening ear and a strong thumb are generally all that is needed. Diagnostic tests, such as X-rays, CAT and MRI scans cannot diagnose the source of pain. As already discussed, CAT and MRI scans routinely show abnormalities which are unrelated to the person's pain complaints.

Once a thorough medical history is obtained from the patient suffering from chronic neck and/or head pain and other associated symptoms are discussed (Barré-Lieou Syndrome), a palpatory examination of the posterior head and neck is performed and tender areas are noted. Again, the accuracy in diagnosing the actual pain-producing area is excellent, because the physician recreates the patient's pain by palpating the neck and posterior head carefully until a positive "jump sign" is elicited. This gives the patient and the physician confidence that the pain-producing structure is between the physician's thumb and the underlying bone. The structure that is typically involved is the cervical vertebral ligaments. These tender areas are treated with Prolotherapy injections. Typical areas treated during a Prolotherapy session for chronic headaches and neck pain are the base of the skull, cervical vertebral ligaments, posterior-lateral clavicle, where the trapezius muscle attaches, as well as the attachment of the levator scapulae muscle. (**Figure 8-6**) Because there is an anesthetic in the solution, generally the neck or headache pain is immediately relieved. This, again, confirms the diagnosis both for the patient and the physician.

Dr. Hackett reported good to excellent results in 90 percent of 82 consecutive patients he treated with neck and/or headache pain.[7,8] Dr. Kayfetz and associates treated 206 patients who had headaches caused from trauma. They found that Prolotherapy was effective in completely relieving the headaches in 79 percent of patients.[9] John Merriman, M.D., of Tulsa, Oklahoma, reported at the 1995 Hackett Foundation Prolotherapy Conference, that in treating the necks of 225 patients with Prolotherapy, 80 percent had good to excellent results.[10] These studies did not differentiate between the different types of headaches. Prolotherapy is effective against migraine, cluster, and tension headaches if ligament laxity is present.

There are several possible reasons why the cure rate is not even higher. Tension headache, also called muscle-contraction headache, affects at least 80 percent of the world's population.[11] It is a problem principally of adult life, with women affected three times as often as men. Aching or squeezing discomfort is typically bilateral in the occiput (base of the skull) or the frontotemporal muscle mass (temple area). There is often also an aching in the base of the neck. This typically occurs because of the head position we all subject ourselves to every day. Whether as a computer operator typing at the terminal, a cook cutting up carrots, or a surgeon performing an operation, the head-forward neck-bent posture stretches the cervical ligaments and the posterior neck muscles, including the levator scapulae and trapezeii. (*As seen in Figure 8-3.*)

Prolotherapy controls the pain of muscle-contraction headache and neck pain. Prolotherapy, however, will not overcome poor posture or poor dietary and lifestyle habits. If a person is continually sleep deprived, stressed out, nutritionally starved (a coffee and doughnut diet), and types on a computer all day, no amount of Prolotherapy will cure that person's neck aches. The cure begins with a proper diet, adequate rest, appropriate stress management, and proper ergonomics at the work station. If pain persists after the above measures are taken, most assuredly a positive response from Prolotherapy treatment will be experienced.

TMJ Syndrome

Another reason a person may not respond adequately to Prolotherapy is that some of the affected areas may not have been treated. A common area forgotten in headache and neck pain is the temporomandibular joint. The temporomandibular joint (TMJ) is the physical connection where the jaw meets the skull. The TMJ is necessary to keep the jaw in proper alignment, especially when talking and eating. A painful and clicking TMJ is called Temporomandibular Joint Syndrome (TMJS). TMJS symptoms are essentially the same as Barré-Leiou Syndrome. It is my belief that the symptoms, such as dizziness, vertigo, etc. that physicians ascribe to the TMJS, are actually due to Barré-Lieou Syndrome.

Causes of TMJ Syndrome

It is well-known that there is a relationship between head posture and jaw

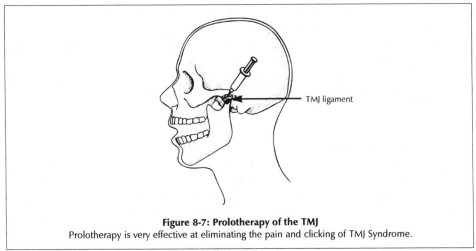

Figure 8-7: Prolotherapy of the TMJ
Prolotherapy is very effective at eliminating the pain and clicking of TMJ Syndrome.

Ligament and Tendon Relaxation Treated by Prolotherapy © 1991, Gustav A. Hemwall, M.D. Used with permission.

position. This can easily be shown by a person putting the head in proper alignment. This position will be comfortable if the lower jaw is back. If the lower jaw is forced forward while the neck and head are in the position, tension is felt in the back of the neck.

Typically in TMJS the lower jaw (mandible) is extended forward. A head forward posture exaggerates the problem.[12,13] This forward mandible aggravates the cervical ligament laxity which increases the neck pain. Again an endless cycle of pain and disability is created in the neck, head, and face region. Prolotherapy injections to strengthen both the cervical vertebrae and the temporomandibular joint will solve this problem. **(Figure 8-7)**

Eventually the mandible moves forward to the extent that it will stretch the lateral TMJ ligament and produce pain. Once the lateral TMJ ligament becomes lax the joint will click. It is important to note that clicking in any joint is an indication of ligament laxity of that joint. Joint clicking is **never** normal or a good sign. Joint clicking, whether it is in the TMJ, knee, neck, or lower back is always abnormal. It is a sign that the bones are beginning to rub against each other. The body's compensatory mechanism for such a situation is to tighten muscles and to grow more bone. The end result will be degeneration, arthritis, and stiffness in that joint. Prolotherapy can stop this process. Prolotherapy will stop a joint from clicking and stop the arthritic process from continuing.

Another reason why a patient may have a lax TMJ ligament is a person's sleeping position. For example, if a patient sleeps with his or her head turned to the right, the TMJ on the left side will be continually stretched throughout the night. Over many decades, continually sleeping in this manner, puts the left TMJ at risk for TMJ ligament laxity. The person with a TMJ problem is advised to sleep with the head turned to the side of the problematic TMJ.

The worst case of TMJS to come into the office was a man I will call T.W. T.W.'s jaw popped so loud that the action of opening his mouth could be heard in the other room. The first Prolotherapy session to his TMJ caused a 60 percent reduction in the clicking of his jaw. After the second treatment, the clicking was eliminated completely. T.W. told me his dentist was amazed. Most dentists and oral surgeons believe TMJ Syndrome is permanent and the best hope is for temporary symptom relief. I can verify in my own practice that TMJ Syndrome can be cured with Prolotherapy. By the way, did the dentist call me to find out what I did? No, they never do.

Treatment of TMJ Syndrome

Louis Schultz, M.D., an oral surgeon, reported in 1956 that, after 20 years of experience in treating hypermobile temporomandibular joints with Prolotherapy, the clicking, grating, or popping was controlled in all of the several thousand patients that had been under his care, without any reported complications or deleterious effects.[14,15] Dr. Schultz wrote, "various types of treatment used in the past (for TMJ Syndrome) and still employed by some operators appear to be unsatisfactory. Surgery is one." One problem with surgery is the resultant scars. Anywhere surgery is done, scar tissue will form. Again, as in all chronic painful conditions, there are a myriad of treatment options. A treatment that includes a surgeon's knife should be reserved until all conservative treatment options have been exhausted.

Prolotherapy in the TMJ is very simple. One to two cc's of a mixture of 25 percent Dextrose, 20 percent Sarapin, and 0.4 percent Lidocaine is injected into and around the temporomandibular joint(s). The patient is placed on a soft diet until the mouth is able to fully open. The TMJ Prolotherapy injections cause an awkward bite and a tight jaw for a couple of days. The patient should not force the mouth open during this time period. Generally, this is an excellent time to start a diet since most people with chronic pain have a positive "basketball-belly sign."

Modern medical practitioners will pressure sick people to utilize their services. Options now available for people with head and neck pain are TMJ arthroscopic surgery, TMJ implants, cervical spine surgery (many varieties), botulinum toxin injections into muscles,[16] and the latest gizmo, surgical cauterization, which zaps the bones with a radiofrequency wave destroying the treated area.[17] This last technique may eliminate a patient's pain because it destroys the fibro-osseous junction, where the pain originates. Why destroy or remove a structure when there is a treatment that will help strengthen and repair it? Prolotherapy causes a permanent strengthening of ligaments and tendons and eliminates the root cause of the pain.

EAR AND MOUTH PAIN

Eagle Syndrome and Ernest Syndrome

One of my patients, J.M., told me, "I have been to a hundred doctors and all I get is a hundred different creams. I am drowning in creams, drops, and pills." Some doctors tell him that the problem is in his ear, others say the ear is fine.

J.M., like many others, suffers from terrible ear and mouth pain. Various diagnoses are typically given for such complaints including otitis media, otitis externa (ear infections), trigeminal neuralgia, atypical facial pain, or TMJ Syndrome. These

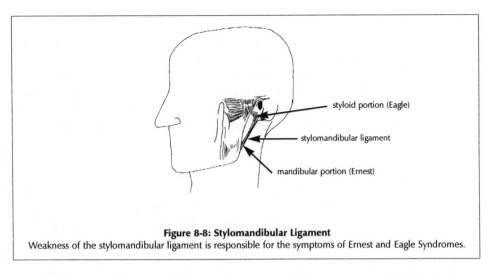

Figure 8-8: Stylomandibular Ligament
Weakness of the stylomandibular ligament is responsible for the symptoms of Ernest and Eagle Syndromes.

diagnoses may be accurate for some; however, chronic unresolved ear, mouth, face, temple, or head pain generally has a ligament laxity etiology. Instead of creams, drops, or pills, J.M. needed a physician to press on his stylomandibular ligament. Most likely he would jump off the table in pain. Chronic pain must be reproduced in the doctor's office to properly diagnose the source of the problem, and thereby provide appropriate treatment.

The stylomandibular ligament originates at the styloid process underneath the ear and inserts on the medial side of the mandible (the lower jaw). **(Figure 8-8)** Pain from the styloid portion of the ligament is called Eagle Syndrome.[18,19] Pain from the mandibular portion is called Ernest Syndrome.[20,21]

The following symptoms have been described with both Eagle and Ernest Syndromes.[22,23]

• Facial pain	• Pain on swallowing	• Voice alteration
• Ear pain	• Pain upon opening the mouth	• Cough
• Forehead pain	• Pain upon turning the head	• Dizziness
• Vertigo	• Difficult jaw opening	• Sinusitis
• TMJ pain	• Mouth pain	• Tinnitus
• Tooth pain	• Throat pain	• Stuffy nose
• Eye pain	• Shoulder pain	• Bloodshot eyes
• Jaw pain	• Excessive lacrimation (tearing)	• Neck pain

Most physicians have not heard of these syndromes and do not know where the stylomandibular ligament is located. For this reason, many people with the above complaints do not obtain relief from their pain. If the diagnosis is wrong, obviously the treatments the physician prescribes will be ineffective.

The stylomandibular and lateral TMJ ligaments attach the jaw to the head. Abnormal motion, excessive movement, or trauma to the jaw may weaken these ligaments. For example, those of us who talk a mile a minute may be prone to TMJ, Eagle, or Ernest Syndromes.

If someone chronically experiences any one of the above symptoms, the stylo-mandibular ligament must be palpated. If a positive "jump sign" can be elicited, the culprit for the chronic ear-mouth pain has most likely been located. Prolotherapy injections at the stylomandibular ligament bony attachments will start the repair process. Once the stylomandibular ligament is strengthened, the chronic ear-mouth pain, tinnitus, dizziness, vertigo, and other pain complaints subside. This is why many people with chronic facial complaints are choosing to Prolo their pain away.

SUMMARY

Chronic headaches, including migraines, neck, temporomandibular joint, ear, and mouth pain originate from ligament laxity in the head, neck, and TMJ. Prolotherapy strengthens the weakened ligaments to relieve the pain. Research has demonstrated that Prolotherapy eliminates 80 to 90 percent of chronic headaches and neck pain. Migraine headaches, as well as other symptoms, including chronic sinus congestion, vertigo, tinnitus, and dysethesias in the arms may be due to Barré-Lieou Syndrome. Prolotherapy permanently strengthens the cervical ligaments and eliminates the Barré-Lieou Syndrome and its symptoms. Prolotherapy is an extremely effective treatment for chronic neck, head, TMJ, facial, ear, and mouth pain because it strengthens the structures that are causing the pain. This is why many people are choosing to Prolo their pain away!

CHAPTER 9

Prolo Your Shoulder Pain Away

T he shoulder was uniquely designed by God to have tremendous mobility. The shoulder enables a person to scratch the head, between the shoulder blades, and even the back without pivoting anything but the shoulder. The lack of big ligamentous structures supporting this joint allow its mobility. The shoulder, when abducted and externally rotated, is more vulnerable to injury due to a lack of bony and ligamentous stability in this position. The primary support for the shoulder involves the rotator cuff muscles that also move the shoulder. People who frequently abduct and externally rotate their shoulders, especially athletes such as pitchers, gymnasts, tennis players, quarterbacks, swimmers, and volleyball players, are prone to chronic shoulder problems. Any activity done with the hand away from the body involves some sort of shoulder abduction and external rotation.[1] **(Figures 9-1)**

A shoulder that crunches and "pops out of joint" is unstable, and is always a sign of weakness in the joint. People who suffer from this condition will feel their shoulder coming out of the socket when they abduct and externally rotate it because the ligamentous and bony support of the joint is minimal in this position. When this occurs, a person is said to have shoulder subluxation or instability. This diagnosis can be confirmed by abducting and externally rotating the shoulder and pushing the arm forward from the back. In the case of anterior shoulder instability, a positive "frighten sign" (the cousin of the infamous positive "jump sign") will be displayed on the patient's face; the patient is afraid his or her shoulder is going to dislocate.

CAUSE AND TREATMENT OF SHOULDER INSTABILITY

Traditional treatment for shoulder instability is rotator cuff strengthening exercises, specifically of the supraspinatus muscle, the primary muscle responsible for the external rotation of the shoulder. The rotator cuff is a group of four muscles: the supraspinatus, infraspinatus, subscapularis, and teres minor. **(Figure 9-2)** The rotator cuff muscles help stabilize the shoulder and assist with movement. Rotator cuff strengthening exercises help strengthen shoulder muscles but often do not cure the underlying problem of shoulder instability: joint laxity.

To cure shoulder joint instability, the ligamentous and shoulder capsular structures must be strengthened. The main capsular structure involved in the stability of the shoulder is the glenoid labrum which holds the humerus bone to the glenoid cavity of the scapula. **(Figure 9-3)** A shoulder is usually unstable because the structures are torn

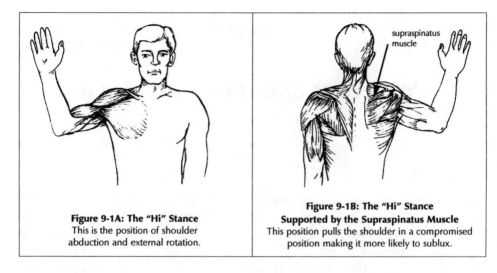

Figure 9-1A: The "Hi" Stance
This is the position of shoulder
abduction and external rotation.

**Figure 9-1B: The "Hi" Stance
Supported by the Supraspinatus Muscle**
This position pulls the shoulder in a compromised
position making it more likely to sublux.

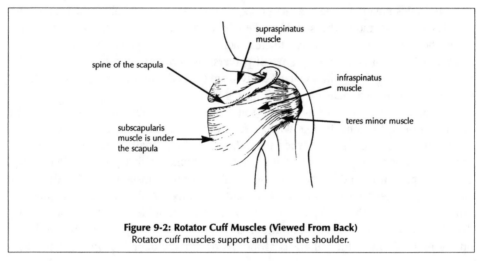

Figure 9-2: Rotator Cuff Muscles (Viewed From Back)
Rotator cuff muscles support and move the shoulder.

or stretched. Another important structure to note in Figure 9-3 is the glenohumeral ligament. Once these structures are stretched or loosened, no amount of exercise will strengthen the shoulder joint enough to permanently hold it in place.

Shoulder instability is one of the easiest conditions to treat with Prolotherapy. Gustav A. Hemwall, M.D., the world's most experienced Prolotherapist, who treated thousands of such cases with Prolotherapy, has never had a pain patient with chronic shoulder instability require surgery. All cases treated with Prolotherapy have recovered without any shoulder limitations, as long as the condition was due to ligament laxity. I have had a similar experience. I have found that even patients with complete shoulder dislocations have fully recovered after being treated with Prolotherapy and have returned to normal activities, including competitive sports, such as tennis, football, baseball, and volleyball.

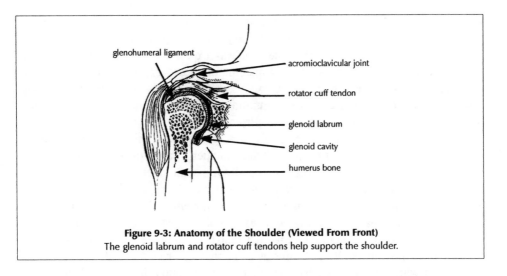

Figure 9-3: Anatomy of the Shoulder (Viewed From Front)
The glenoid labrum and rotator cuff tendons help support the shoulder.

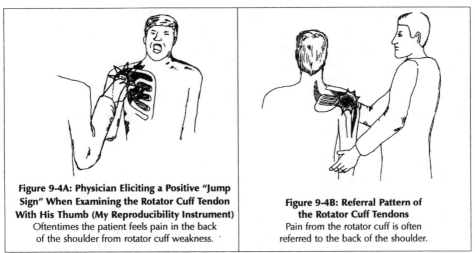

Figure 9-4A: Physician Eliciting a Positive "Jump Sign" When Examining the Rotator Cuff Tendon With His Thumb (My Reproducibility Instrument)
Oftentimes the patient feels pain in the back of the shoulder from rotator cuff weakness.

Figure 9-4B: Referral Pattern of the Rotator Cuff Tendons
Pain from the rotator cuff is often referred to the back of the shoulder.

ROTATOR CUFF TENDONITIS

The most common cause of chronic shoulder pain, however, is not shoulder instability, but supraspinatus tendon weakness, also known as rotator cuff tendonitis.[2,3] As noted, the ligamentous, capsular, and bony support of the shoulder in the abducted and externally rotated position is minimal, so the supraspinatus tendon works harder to provide support. The supraspinatus tendon eventually weakens and laxity develops. A supraspinatus tendon problem is manifested by pain with abduction and external rotation of the shoulder, especially when reaching for things above shoulder level, or pain in the shoulder after sleeping due to compression of the supraspinatus tendon. The supraspinatus tendon often refers pain to the back of the shoulder. **(Figures 9-4)** The supraspinatus tendon is the main abductor and external rotator of the shoulder. Sleeping on the shoulder causes a pinching of the rotator cuff muscles and can lead to rotator cuff weakness. There are cases where the cause of the rotator cuff tendon laxity was due to years of sleeping on the shoulder.

In most cases, traditional therapies such as exercise and physical therapy will resolve rotator cuff tendonitis. It is not uncommon, however, for rotator cuff injuries to linger because blood supply to the rotator cuff tendons is poor.[4] Poor blood supply is a reason the rotator cuff is so commonly injured. In chronic cases of shoulder pain due to rotator cuff weakness, Prolotherapy is the treatment of choice. Prolotherapy will cause the rotator cuff to strengthen and eliminate shoulder pain. If rotator cuff weakness is not corrected, the shoulder's range of motion will deteriorate. Rapid deterioration can occur, especially in people over 60 years of age.

As previously stated, the supraspinatus muscle causes shoulder abduction and external rotation. When this muscle weakens, movement becomes painful. Those who have supraspinatus tendon laxity causing pain will stop moving their arms into the painful position. Though they may not realize it, they are slowly but surely losing shoulder movement. What begins as a simple rotator cuff muscle weakness easily treated with Prolotherapy, has the potential to become a frozen shoulder because of scar tissue formation inside the shoulder that was left untreated. The scar tissue formation causing a decrease in the ability to move the shoulder is called adhesive capsulitis. Pain means something is wrong. Prolotherapy, because it eliminates the cause of most chronic pain, should be tried before a complication of the pain occurs, as seen in the above example.

What began as a simple rotator cuff tendon weakness easily treated with Prolotherapy has turned into adhesive capsulitis, or frozen shoulder, a much more challenging condition to treat due to the scar tissue formation.

FROZEN SHOULDER (ADHESIVE CAPSULITIS)

A frozen shoulder is also treatable with Prolotherapy, but healing occurs over a longer period of time. The term adhesive capsulitis refers to scar tissue that forms inside the joint due to lack of movement. If a joint is not moved through its full range of motion every day, scar tissue will form inside the joint. Adhesive capsulitis is especially common in stroke victims who are paralyzed on one side because they are unable to move their shoulders through a full range of motion.[5]

The first line of treatment for a frozen shoulder is physiotherapy. Physical therapy modalities such as myofascial release, massage, range-of-motion exercises, and ultrasound can often release scar tissue. If these do not relieve the problem, then the scar tissue can be broken up within the joint by the physician injecting the shoulder full of a solution made up of sterile water mixed with an anesthetic. The numb shoulder can then be gently manipulated. Often several sessions of this treatment regime are needed to achieve the shoulder's original full range-of-motion.

Since the initial cause of the adhesive capsulitis was supraspinatus (rotator cuff) weakness, Prolotherapy injections to strengthen the rotator cuff are done in conjunction with the above technique. Complete to near-complete resolution can be accomplished using this combined approach.

A misunderstanding of the supraspinatus tendon's referral pattern keeps clinicians

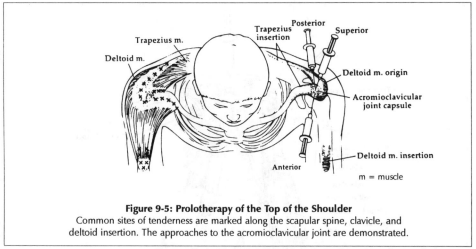

Figure 9-5: Prolotherapy of the Top of the Shoulder
Common sites of tenderness are marked along the scapular spine, clavicle, and deltoid insertion. The approaches to the acromioclavicular joint are demonstrated.

Ligament and Tendon Relaxation Treated by Prolotherapy © 1991, Gustav A. Hemwall, M.D. Used with permission.

from diagnosing the rotator cuff problem. This tendon refers pain to the back and side of the shoulder leading clinicians to believe their patients have a muscle problem, when in fact they have a tendon problem. A complaint of shoulder pain is almost always a rotator cuff weakness problem. Prolotherapy is extremely effective at strengthening the rotator cuff tendons.

ACROMIOCLAVICULAR JOINT/CORACOID PROCESS

Another common cause of chronic shoulder pain is a weak attachment of the clavicle to the acromion. This joint is called the acromioclavicular joint and is noted on the surface of the skin at the apex (top) of the shoulder. (**Figure 9-5**) This joint is usually injured in a fall or by a hyperextension of the shoulder.[6] When this occurs, the weight of the body is transmitted to the acromioclavicular joint. This joint, like all joints, is held together by ligaments. When these ligaments are injured and become lax, the joint grinds and grates and causes pain. Acromioclavicular ligament laxity causes pain upon lifting or activity involving the hands in front or across the body. Prolotherapy is extremely effective at strengthening the acromioclavicular ligaments, eliminating the shoulder grinding and chronic shoulder pain from this area.

A lesser known cause of shoulder pain emanates from the coracoid process. From this little nub of bone stem some very important structures including, the pectoralis minor muscle, coracobrachialis muscle, biceps muscle, coracoacromial ligament, coracoclavicular ligament, coracohumeral ligament, and parts of the articular capsule. All attach on a nub of bone no bigger than the tip of the little finger. Though small, this area is "mighty" in regards to importance. This area of the shoulder is palpated during a routine Prolotherapy shoulder examination. Chronic shoulder pain patients are typically very tender in this area and a positive "jump sign" can be elicited upon palpation. Prolotherapy injections are given to strengthen the fibro-osseous junctions of all the above structures at the coracoid process. (**Figure 9-6**) This area is routinely treated to relieve chronic shoulder pain.

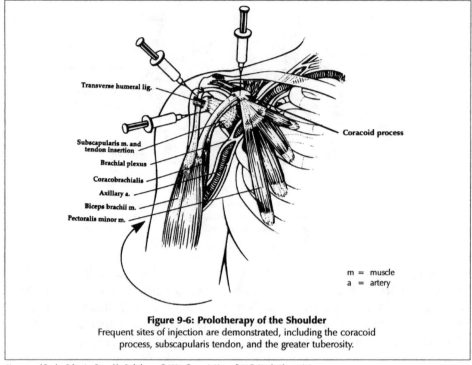

Figure 9-6: Prolotherapy of the Shoulder
Frequent sites of injection are demonstrated, including the coracoid
process, subscapularis tendon, and the greater tuberosity.

IMPINGEMENT SYNDROME

Approximately five percent of patients with chronic shoulder pain do not find relief from Prolotherapy injections. These people usually have Impingement Syndrome. This is caused by the supraspinatus tendon being pinched between the coracohumeral ligament, from the clavicle above, and the humerus below. People often have a bony spur on the clavicle that decreases the space through which the supraspinatus tendon must travel.[7]

Occasionally, surgery is needed to give the supraspinatus tendon more room to move. (Like me, it needs its own space.) The diagnosis can be easily confirmed in the office by observing a grimaced and painful face upon abducting and internally rotating the shoulder producing a positive "impingement sign." **(Figure 9-7)** It should be noted that even with an initial diagnosis of Impingement Syndrome, the majority of people obtain complete or satisfactory relief of their pain with Prolotherapy alone. In the few patients who have needed surgery for Impingement Syndrome after Prolotherapy, the response rate of the combined approach has been excellent. The Prolotherapy has strengthened the rotator cuff tendons and surgery has eliminated the impingement of those tendons, leading to complete relief of the chronic shoulder pain.

PROLOTHERAPY FOR SHOULDER PAIN

Prolotherapy will cause the growth of the rotator cuff tendons whether or not they are torn, stretched, or pinched as described above. Prolotherapy causes the

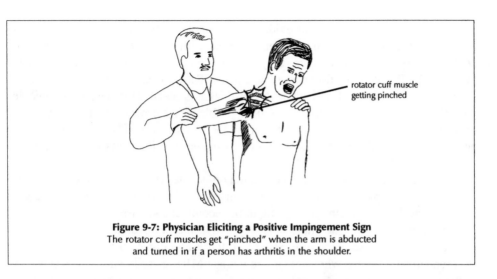

Figure 9-7: Physician Eliciting a Positive Impingement Sign
The rotator cuff muscles get "pinched" when the arm is abducted
and turned in if a person has arthritis in the shoulder.

growth of any ligament, tendon, capsule, or muscle tissue at the fibro-osseous junction. Prolotherapy is ineffective only if there has been a complete tear of the ligament or tendon. In such cases, surgery must be performed. However, 98 percent of all chronic pain cases do not involve complete ligament and tendon tears, and Prolotherapy is the treatment of choice.

It is always worthwhile to have an evaluation by a physician skilled in Prolotherapy prior to any surgical procedure for pain. Physicians who utilize Prolotherapy in their practice understand ligament referral patterns and are skilled in diagnosing ligament and tendon relaxation. In more than 95 percent of cases, surgery performed simply on the basis of chronic pain can be avoided by using Prolotherapy.

UNRELIABILITY OF MRI FOR DIAGNOSIS OF LIGAMENT INJURY

Many researchers have shown that X-ray studies of the shoulder often do not reveal the source of the problem, as abnormal MRI results are often seen in patients with no shoulder pain symptoms.[8,9,10] Vijay Chandnani, M.D., and associates, presented results of a study involving people 25 to 55 years of age who were asymptomatic. The following were the findings from their MRI scans of the shoulder: 35 percent had bone spurs of the acromioclavicular joint, 35 percent had evidence of rotator cuff pathology, and 50 percent had abnormalities in the glenoid labrum.[11] C. Neumann, M.D., and associates, examined 55 asymptomatic shoulders with T1-weighted MRI scans and showed that 89 percent had abnormalities in the supraspinatus tendon.[12] I find it incredible that 89 percent of people have abnormalities in their rotator cuff tendons on MRI even though they have no symptoms whatsoever!

The most recent study conducted by Jerry Sher, M.D., and associates, published in 1995, examined MRI scans of 96 people who had no symptoms of shoulder pain. This study revealed that 34 percent of the individuals showed a partial tear of the rotator cuff and 15 percent had evidence of complete full-thickness tears. This is obviously an erroneous reading because people with complete tears of the rotator cuff would not be asymptomatic: they would not be able to move their shoulders much at all. People over 60 years of age had MRI scans showing 54 percent with rotator cuff tears and 28 percent with full-thickness tears. This means that people over 60 years of age without any shoulder problems whatsoever have a 54 percent chance of the MRI scan showing a tear of the rotator cuff. They also have a 28 percent chance of the MRI scan showing a complete full-thickness tear of the rotator cuff.[13]

Remember, these studies were conducted on people who did not have any symptoms of shoulder pain. If someone goes to an orthopedic surgeon for chronic shoulder pain, guess what treatment is going to be recommended based on the MRI scan? You guessed it! Sliced shoulder! It is imperative that an evaluation be done by a Prolotherapist because diagnostic tests can often lead a clinician astray.

I remember a patient who came to me with an MRI scan showing a complete tear of the rotator cuff. Upon physical examination of this patient, it was evident that the tear was not complete. After several sessions of Prolotherapy, the patient's shoulder was symptom-free. There is no substitute for a listening ear and a strong thumb. If physicians cannot reproduce their patient's pain in the office, they probably cannot get rid of it either. A Prolotherapist can reproduce a patient's pain using his or her own MRI (**M**y **R**eproducibility **I**nstrument, the thumb) and can eliminate the pain. Reproduction of pain by a good physical examination, combined with elimination of the pain by Prolotherapy, is far more effective in diagnosing the cause of chronic shoulder pain than any CAT or MRI scan. (*See Figures 9-4.*)

SUMMARY

Chronic shoulder pain is usually due to a weakness in the rotator cuff, specifically in the supraspinatus tendon, because the tendon has poor blood supply. If left untreated, this supraspinatus tendon laxity leads to adhesive capsulitis or frozen shoulder. Other common reasons for chronic shoulder pain are acromioclavicular ligament laxity, shoulder instability due to a weakened glenohumeral ligament or glenoid labrum tear, and weakness of the structures that attach to the coracoid process.

MRI scans of the shoulder are often abnormal in individuals without any shoulder symptoms whatsoever. The best diagnostic procedure for chronic shoulder pain is palpation of the structure causing a positive "jump sign" and relief of the pain immediately after the structure is treated with Prolotherapy. Prolotherapy is the treatment of choice for chronic shoulder pain because it corrects the underlying weakness causing the pain. This is why many people are choosing to Prolo their shoulder pain away.

CHAPTER 10

Prolo Your Elbow, Wrist, and Hand Pain Away

B ecause of our modern high-tech society, many people sit all day looking at a computer screen and typing on a keyboard. Some children in first and second grades are required to do their schoolwork on a computer. I am not against technology, but I don't think man was made to punch little buttons several hundred thousand times per day.

Typically people who perform repetitive tasks with their hands are the patients with chronic elbow, wrist, and hand pain.[1] This includes mail handlers, assembly line workers, carpenters, computer operators, secretaries, and the thousands of other jobs that keep people in one space doing the same thing day after day. Is it any wonder that after repeating a movement 10 billion times that a part of the body breaks down?

After a long hard day of work or strenuous exercise, it is quite normal for muscles to hurt for a short period of time. This is often a "good hurt." You worked hard and deserve to have your spouse rub your feet. (But how many of them do?) The muscles ache after a good workout because muscle cells were actually injured during exercise. Yes, you read that correctly. Exercise and repetitive work does cause injury to muscle cells. But such injury is good for the muscles because they have a tremendous blood supply and this "temporary injury" stimulates muscle cells to multiply and grow. If you exercise daily, new blood vessels form and soon you may be as "studly" as Arnold Schwarzenegger.

God made muscles with the ability to be ready for a fight. It is a necessary defense mechanism that, at a moment's notice, the blood supply to our muscles can increase tenfold. If you wake up to find that your house is on fire, the blood supply to the muscles can increase to give them the strength to rescue you. Exercise is necessary for good health and keeps the muscles strong.

This "good hurt" with exercise should not last more than an hour or two. If the muscles hurt longer than this time period, you are either exercising too much or need to take more breaks during work.

An extreme case of overexertion was my running in the Chicago Marathon in 1988. I knew I would be a little stiff after the race so I planned to take the following week as vacation. Prior to the race, 16 miles was my longest run. I ran the race with my buddy, Glenn, who had already finished several marathons.

Unfortunately for me, the day of the race was too cold for anyone other than

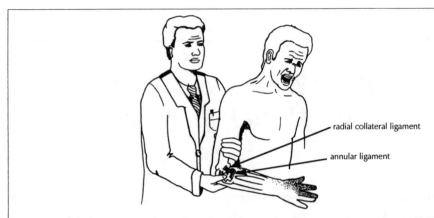

Figure 10-1: Physician Palpates the Annular Ligament, Eliciting the Referral Pain Pattern Down the Arm
Weakness in the annular ligament refers pain to the thumb and the index and middle fingers.

polar bears. Four hours and eight minutes after I started off, I crossed the finish line a winner. Yes, a winner. I was told at the end of the race, "to run is to win." However, for the next five days I felt like a loser. I felt nauseated, stiff, achy, extremely hot, and totally drained. No amount of massage, ice, heat, or tender loving care (This almost always works.) could make me feel well after that "exercise." Fortunately, I was eventually able to walk again!

Many people attempt similar feats of stardom on the weekends. They are known as weekend warriors. A good example of a weekend warrior is my friend, Kurt. At least once a month, he injures himself doing some sporting event. Kurt somehow thinks that sitting at a desk all day is training enough to become Karch Karaly on the volleyball court during the weekend. The main point is to exercise at a level consistent with your lifestyle. If your main exercise during the week is getting up from the couch, putting down the remote, and going to the kitchen to get ice cream from the freezer, it is not wise to play in a basketball league on weekends.

Muscle injuries usually heal with plain and simple rest. To speed up recovery from muscle injuries, it is beneficial to stretch the muscles after exercising.[2] Nutritional supplements also help muscle injuries heal.[3] (*See Appendix A, Nutrition and Chronic Pain, and Appendix C, Natural Medicine Resources.*)

Chronic pain that is not relieved by rest is likely due to a ligament injury. Pain with repetitive motion may be an indication of tendon injury. Ligaments attach bone to bone. While the ligaments stabilize the bones, the tendons and muscles enable the bones to move. This is why ligaments often hurt when the body is at rest and tendons often hurt from activity.

ELBOW PAIN
Annular Ligament Weakness

Eighty percent of chronic elbow pain is due to a sprain of the annular ligament. **(Figure 10-1)** This ligament is rarely examined by a family physician or an orthopedic surgeon. Nearly all of my patients with chronic elbow pain tell me their doctors told them they have tennis elbow. Tennis elbow is also known as lateral epicondylitis. The latest treatment for this condition is the dreaded cortisone shot! Cortisone weakens tissue, whereas Prolotherapy strengthens tissue. Cortisone has temporary effects in regard to pain control whereas Prolotherapy has permanent effects. However, cortisone does have one permanent effect: Continual use will permanently weaken tissue. Anyone receiving long-term prednisone or cortisone shots will confirm this fact.

The annular ligament is located approximately three quarters of an inch distal to the lateral epicondyle. Its job is to attach the radius bone to the ulnar bone. It is this ligament that enables the hand to rotate, as in turning a key or a screwdriver. Because of the tremendous demands placed on the fingers and hands to perform repetitive tasks, the annular ligament is stressed every day. (Like a lot of people I know.) Eventually, this ligament becomes lax and a source of chronic pain.

The lateral epicondyle of the humerus bone is very superficial so it is much more inviting to the dreaded cortisone-filled needle of an orthopedist than the deeper annular ligament. Typically, people with chronic elbow pain are tender over the lateral epicondyle, but do not elicit a positive "jump sign" in that area. Only palpation over the annular ligament elicits the positive "jump sign." The annular ligament also has a distinct referral pain pattern. It refers pain to the thumb, index, and middle fingers. This is the same referral pain pattern as is exhibited in Carpal Tunnel Syndrome.

Unfortunately, many patients with elbow and hand pain have been mis-diagnosed with Carpal Tunnel Syndrome. Carpal Tunnel Syndrome refers to the entrapment of the median nerve as it travels through the wrist into the hand. The nerve supplies sensation to the skin over the thumb, index, and middle fingers. A typical Carpal Tunnel Syndrome patient will experience pain and numbness in this distribution in the hand. Because most physicians do not know the referral pain patterns of ligaments, they do not realize that cervical vertebrae 4 and 5 and the annular ligament can refer pain to the thumb, index, and middle fingers. Ligament laxity can also cause numbness, as already discussed. Cervical and annular ligament laxity should always be evaluated prior to making the diagnosis of Carpal Tunnel Syndrome. Surgery for Carpal Tunnel Syndrome should not be done until an evaluation is performed by a physician who understands the referral patterns of ligaments and is experienced in Prolotherapy.

Seldom do patients find relief from the "Carpal Tunnel" complaints of pain in the hand and elbow with physical therapy and surgery because the diagnosis is wrong. The most common reason for pain in the elbow referring pain to the hand is weakness in the annular ligament, not from Carpal Tunnel Syndrome. Several sessions of Prolotherapy will easily strengthen the annular ligament and relieve chronic elbow pain.

Ulnar Collateral Ligament Weakness

Another common cause of chronic elbow pain is an ulnar collateral ligament sprain. **(Figure 10-2)** This ligament supports the inside of the elbow. It is responsible for holding the ulnar bone to the distal end of the humerus. This enables the arm

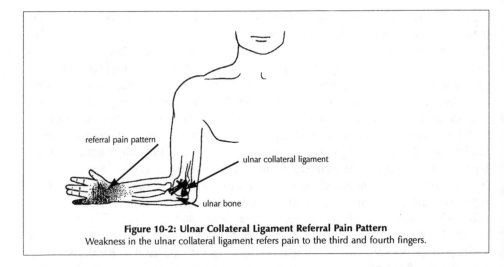

Figure 10-2: Ulnar Collateral Ligament Referral Pain Pattern
Weakness in the ulnar collateral ligament refers pain to the third and fourth fingers.

to flex, pivoting at the elbow. A patient's complaint of pain on the inside of the elbow will cause a physician to examine the lateral epicondyle's "sister," the medial epicondyle. For example, the diagnosing of the golfer's elbow is often made without examining the ulnar collateral ligament.

The ulnar collateral ligament is approximately three quarters of an inch distal to the medial epicondyle. The ulnar collateral ligament refers pain to the little finger and ring finger. This same pain and numbness distribution is seen with aggravating the ulnar nerve. The ulnar nerve lies behind the elbow and is the reason why hitting your funny bone causes pain. Because most physicians are not familiar with the referral pattern of ligaments, patients with elbow pain and/or numbness into the little finger and ring finger are diagnosed with an ulnar nerve problem, Cubital Tunnel Syndrome. A more common reason is ligament laxity in the cervical vertebrae 6 and 7 or in the ulnar collateral ligament, not a pinched ulnar nerve.

As stated, a patient given the opinion that surgery on the ulnar nerve is needed for a pain complaint should obtain a second opinion from a doctor who is competent in the treatment of Prolotherapy. Surgery should be performed only after all conservative options, including Prolotherapy, have been attempted. Prolotherapy to the ulnar collateral ligament is the most successful way to eliminate medial elbow pain.

If medial epicondylitis (golfer's elbow) or lateral epicondylitis (tennis elbow) is causing elbow pain, the muscles that attach to these areas are attempting to repair themselves, causing inflammation. The treatment should not be to "anti-inflame," as is the case with cortisone or with anti-inflammatories like ibuprofen. The correct treatment is to strengthen the muscle attachments which are inflamed due to the body's attempt to strengthen the area. The muscles that extend the wrist attach at the lateral epicondyle and the muscles that flex the wrist attach at the medial epicondyle. Prolotherapy to strengthen these muscle attachments is very effective in eliminating chronic elbow pain.

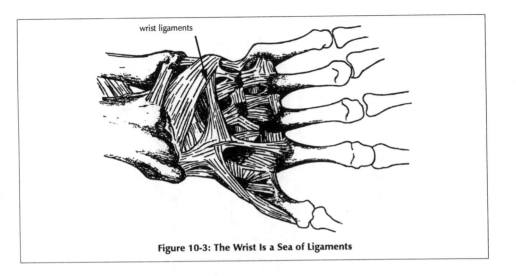

Figure 10-3: The Wrist Is a Sea of Ligaments

WRIST PAIN

Weakened ligaments commonly cause chronic wrist pain. The weakened ligaments allow one of the eight wrist bones to become unstable and shift positions. This condition is called carpal instability. The wrist is actually eight oddly shaped bones in a sea of ligaments.[4] **(Figure 10-3)** The most common wrist bones that become unstable because of loose ligaments are the capitate, scaphoid, and lunate.[5,6] Thus, the most common ligaments treated with Prolotherapy for chronic wrist pain are the dorsal capitate-trapezoid, hamate-capitate, scaphoid-triquetral, and scapholunate ligaments. Again, the diagnosis is easily made by direct palpation of these ligaments, as the wrist bones are very superficial to the skin. The weakened ligament can be palpated and a positive "jump sign" elicited. Several Prolotherapy sessions in this area resolves the problem.

A few points need to be made about bony alignment and the role of Prolotherapy. Prolotherapy injections strengthen the ligaments which attach to the bones. The ligaments, after returning to normal strength, will produce proper bone alignment. Patients who are under the care of a chiropractor, in addition to a Prolotherapy physician, often comment that their chiropractor is amazed by how well the spine has moved into alignment.

Remember, Prolotherapy is an effective treatment for any structural pain problem that involves a weak ligament or tendon. Regardless of the area of the body involved, four Prolotherapy sessions are usually all that is needed to resolve the chronic pain problem in a healthy individual.

HAND PAIN

When it comes to hand pain, the most common problem involves the thumb because of its unique role in the hand's function. Whenever a doorknob is turned, a screwdriver is used, or something is held, the thumb is part of the action. When typing, what part of the hand must continually hit the space bar? The thumb.

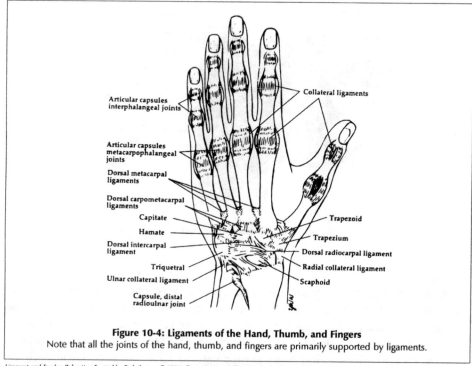

Figure 10-4: Ligaments of the Hand, Thumb, and Fingers
Note that all the joints of the hand, thumb, and fingers are primarily supported by ligaments.

Ligament and Tendon Relaxation Treated by Prolotherapy © 1991, Gustav A. Hemwall, M.D. Used with permission.

Because thumbs have to work so much harder than fingers, it is usually the first to elicit pain. The thumb ligament that joins the wrist to the base of the thumb is called the radial collateral ligament, the same name as the ligament inside the elbow. The thumb ligament that joins the base of the thumb, the first metacarpal, to the succeeding joint, proximal phalanx, is the collateral ligament. **(Figure 10-4)**

These two joints of the thumb, called the carpometacarpal (CMC) and metacarpophalangeal (MCP), are usually the first areas where pain is experienced. If the ligaments in these joints are not strengthened, arthritis will eventually occur. Arthritis starts the day a joint becomes loose. The looser the joint, the greater the chance it has of becoming arthritic. Arthritis in the thumb, as well as other phalangeal joints in the hand, are a major cause of disability, especially among the elderly.[7,8] The progression of osteoarthritis stops the day the ligaments become strong and are able to stabilize the joint. (*See Chapter 14, Prolo Your Arthritis Pain Away.*)

Prolotherapy is the treatment of choice for patients suffering from stiff, sore hands or thumbs. Once the ligaments are strengthened, the pain and stiffness in the thumbs and fingers subside. Again, four Prolotherapy treatment sessions are usually all that is needed.

SUMMARY

Chronic pain in the arms, elbows, wrists, and hands is primarily due to the type of work people perform in a modern high-tech society. The repetitive motions of the upper extremities eventually wear out the ligamentous support of the elbows, wrists, and thumbs. The end result is loose joints that cause pain and stiffness. Prolotherapy injections start the healing process to cause the growth of ligaments that stabilize these joints. Once the ligaments return to normal strength, the chronic pain is eliminated. Because of this, many people with chronic elbow, wrist, and hand pain are choosing to Prolo their pain away.

CHAPTER 11

Prolo Your Groin, Hip, and Knee Pain Away

T he old saying that "the foot bone is connected to the knee bone is connected to the hip bone" sure holds true when it comes to leg and hip pain. To adequately eliminate hip, knee, and leg pain, the entire extremity must be evaluated. As stated in Chapter Seven, the most common cause for low back pain is laxity in the sacroiliac joint. Prolotherapy injections to strengthen the sacroiliac joint eliminates the pain. As usual, the original cause of the sacroiliac ligament laxity must be addressed to ensure long-term pain relief.

In 1911, Ronald Meisenbach, M.D., observed that "individuals with pendulous abdomens are frequently in a state of lipomatosis with very flabby and relaxed ligaments."[1] In common language, flabby bellies lead to flabby sacroiliac ligaments. The more weight that hangs over the belt line, the more stressed the sacroiliac ligaments become. To ensure long-term healing for low back and hip pain, maintenance of a proper weight is encouraged. Dr. Meisenbach also wrote that "it is now beginning to be recognized that almost all of the sciaticas are due to sacroiliac relaxation."[2] This is exactly what Gustav A. Hemwall, M.D., the world's most experienced Prolotherapist, taught me when I was learning Prolotherapy.

GROIN PAIN

Another common cause of chronic hip pain is the Iliolumbar Syndrome.[3] This syndrome is caused by ligament laxity of the iliolumbar ligaments. The common symptoms are not only hip pain, but also pain referred to the groin. (*See Figures 2-2.*) Iliolumbar ligament laxity should be explored as a diagnosis for any patient with unresolved groin pain.

Several years ago, the late David Brewer, M.D., a personal friend and a respected obstetrician/gynecologist, examined a young woman with unresolved lower abdominal/groin pain. The young woman was scheduled for an exploratory laparoscopic surgery to the pelvic region. The possible diagnosis was endometriosis or an ovarian cyst. Interestingly, the surgery had to be postponed until Dr. Brewer returned from a conference. At that conference, Dr. Brewer learned about Prolotherapy and the ligament referral patterns.

When this young woman returned for her pre-surgery physical examination, Dr. Brewer proceeded to examine the iliolumbar ligament. You can guess what happened— a positive "jump sign." He treated the area with Prolotherapy and immediately the chronic lower abdominal and groin pain were gone. Whew! Another surgery prevented! Needless to say, Dr. Brewer became a quick believer in Prolotherapy.

This case illustrates a point that has been made over and over again. Prior to any surgical procedure for pain, it is important to have an evaluation by a physician familiar with Prolotherapy. The main cause of unresolved chronic pain is weakness in a ligament. Surgery does not cause ligaments to regrow but can cause harm and will surely empty your pocketbook.

Chronic groin pain is easily treated with Prolotherapy because there are multiple ligament laxities that cause groin pain. This diagnosis is accomplished by the physician having a listening ear and a strong thumb. An interesting case will illustrate this point.

A young woman came to see me having suffered for more than 10 years with terrible groin pain. She had stepped into an animal trap which wrapped around her leg. This caused the trap to engage and before she knew it, she found herself hanging upside down from a tree limb with the rope lassoed around her ankle. Alone in the forest, she hung there for what seemed like eternity until she was finally rescued. As a result of this incident, she was left with chronic groin and back pain. As a health food store owner, she turned to numerous healing techniques. She also sought relief from many doctors who diagnosed her as having, among other things, a groin sprain, a disc problem, and a tendon strain. Nothing permanently relieved her pain.

Her medical history clearly indicated one thing that could have caused the problem. I compressed the pubic symphysis (the pubic joint ligament) with my thumb on the side of the leg that had been caught in the rope. Wow! That caused a whole body "jump sign." I treated that area with Prolotherapy. For the first time in a decade, she walked without pain.

Only once has a patient told me that a physician had examined the pubic symphysis. The pubic symphysis is the front joint of the pelvic bone. (Figure 11-1) The back joint of the pelvic bone is the sacroiliac joint. If the sacroiliac joint is lax, there is a good chance that the pubic symphysis will also be lax. Regarding the treatment of chronic pain with Prolotherapy, it is advisable to treat both sides of a joint to ensure its strength. Someone suffering from low back pain should not only have the sacroiliac joints examined, but the pubic symphysis as well. Likewise, patients with groin pain should have the sacroiliac joints palpated. Sacroiliac ligament laxity can also refer pain to the groin.[4]

The pubic symphysis is actually a disc. It is a fibrocartilagenous disc that, like any other disc in the body, can be disrupted. It is supported on top by the superior pubic ligaments. Typically, people with groin pain are assumed to have a groin strain. This refers to a strain of the adductor muscles that attach to the pubic bone. (Figure 11-1) Chronic pain that does not respond to exercise, massage, or manipulation is most likely a ligament problem. In the case of pain reproduced by palpating the pubic symphysis, the cause of the pain is pubic symphysis diathesis. This means a loose pubic symphysis area. Unfortunately, mild laxity in the joints can only be diagnosed by palpation. There is no X-ray study that can be done to confirm it. This

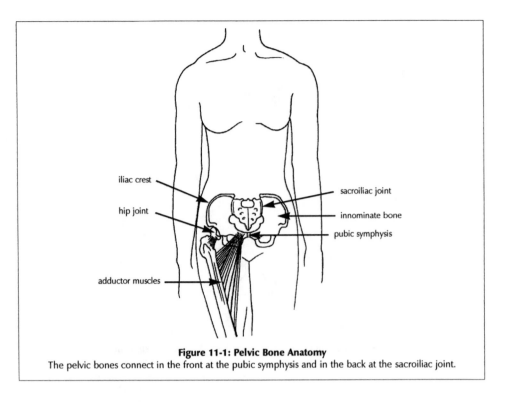

Figure 11-1: Pelvic Bone Anatomy
The pelvic bones connect in the front at the pubic symphysis and in the back at the sacroiliac joint.

is also why many physicians do not diagnose it. The diagnosis of ligament laxity can generally only be made by a listening ear and a strong thumb.

The pubic symphysis joint is stressed when the leg is pulled out from underneath, as in the case of the lassoed lady. This can also be caused by falling, tripping, or slipping. In sports, pubic symphysis injuries are relatively frequent. Swimmers who do the breast stroke often suffer groin pain from a pubic symphysis injury. Prolotherapy for pubic symphysis diathesis entails injections into the fibro-osseous junction of the superior pubic symphysis ligament and injections in the pubic symphysis itself. Prolotherapy is extremely effective in strengthening the pubic symphysis and relieving chronic groin pain in this area.

HIP PAIN

The hip joint joins the leg to the pelvis. Unfortunately, for most people, both legs are not exactly the same. They may look the same, but from a bio-mechanical standpoint, they are not the same. One leg may be rotated either in or out, or one leg may be shorter than the other. The latter is especially common if one leg was broken during childhood. Because the hip joint connects the leg to the pelvis, the hip joint will sustain the brunt of any bio-mechanical abnormality that may occur. If one leg is shorter than the other, the hip joints will be stressed because the leg length discrepancy causes an abnormal gait (manner of walking). The gait cycle is most efficient when the iliac crests (pelvis) are level. Unequal leg lengths cause the

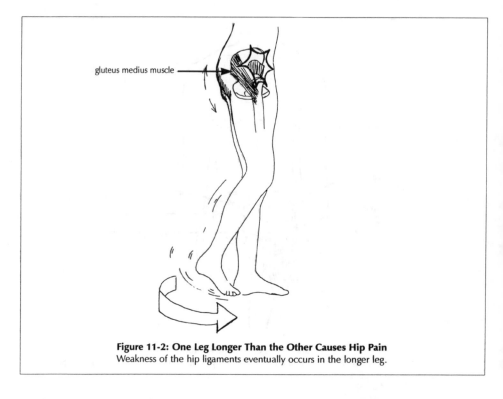

Figure 11-2: One Leg Longer Than the Other Causes Hip Pain
Weakness of the hip ligaments eventually occurs in the longer leg.

pelvis to move abnormally. This is evidenced by the waddling gait of someone with a hip problem. This waddling gait helps remove pressure on the painful hip.

With leg length discrepancy, either hip joint can cause pain and usually both hip joints hurt to some degree.[5] To propel the leg forward, the hip joint must be raised which strains the gluteus medius muscle and the posterior hip ligaments. **(Figure 11-2)** Leg length problems are also associated with recurrent lower back problems because they cause the pelvis to be asymmetric.[6] Prolotherapy to the sacroiliac and hip joints will correct the asymmetries in the majority of cases. The leg length discrepancy disappears from the leveling of the pelvis. If asymmetry remains after treatment, a shoe insert or heel lift will generally correct the problem.

A problem in the hip may commonly manifest itself as groin or inguinal pain. Someone suffering from groin pain should be examined at the pubic symphysis, sacroiliac joint, iliolumbar ligaments, and hip joint. Pain from the hip joint may also be felt locally, directly above the hip joint in the back. When the hip joint becomes lax, the muscles over the joint compensate for the laxity by tensing. As is the case with any joint of the body, lax ligaments initiate muscle tension in an attempt to stabilize the joint. This compensatory mechanism to stabilize the hip joint eventually causes the gluteus medius, muscle pyriformis, and iliotibial band/tensor fascia lata muscles to tighten because of chronic contraction in an attempt to compensate for a loose hip joint. The contracted gluteus medius can eventually irritate the trochanteric bursa causing a trochanteric bursitis. A bursa is a fluid-filled sac which

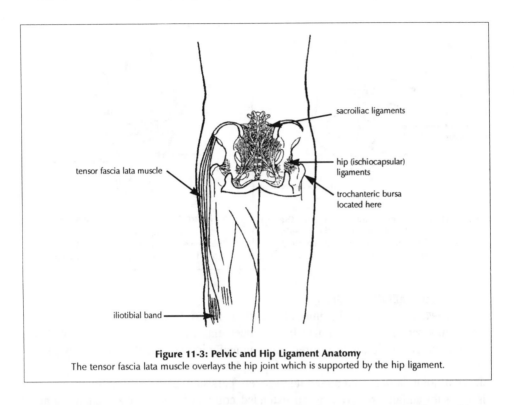

Figure 11-3: Pelvic and Hip Ligament Anatomy
The tensor fascia lata muscle overlays the hip joint which is supported by the hip ligament.

helps muscles glide over bony prominences. Patients with chronic hip problems often have had cortisone injected into this bursa, which generally brings temporary relief. But this treatment does not provide permanent relief because the underlying ligament laxity is not being corrected. Prolotherapy injections to strengthen the hip joint and iliocapsular ligaments will provide definitive relief in such a case.

It is interesting to note that trochanteric bursitis, Pyriformi Syndrome, and weakness in the iliotibial band also cause "sciatica."[7,8] Someone suffering from "sciatica" should request the physician to examine the following structures: sacroiliac joint, hip joint, sacrotuberous and sacrospinous ligaments, trochanteric bursa, and iliotibial band/tensor fascia lata. The sciatic nerve runs between the two heads of the pyriformi muscle. When the pyriformi muscle is spastic, the sciatic nerve may be pinched. Lumbosacral and hip joint weaknesses are two main causes of pyriformi muscle spasm. Pyriformi muscle stretches and physical therapy directed at the pyriformi muscle to reduce spasm help temporarily, but do not alleviate the real problem. Prolotherapy of the hip and lower back strengthens those joints, thus eliminating the pyriformi muscle spasms.

The iliotibial band/tensor fascia lata extends from the pelvis over the hip joint to the lateral knee. **(Figure 11-3)** Its job is to help abduct the leg, especially during walking so the legs do not cross when walking. When this band/muscle is tight, it puts a great strain on the sacroiliac and lumbosacral ligaments.[9] Stretching this muscle is very beneficial to many people with chronic hip/back problems.

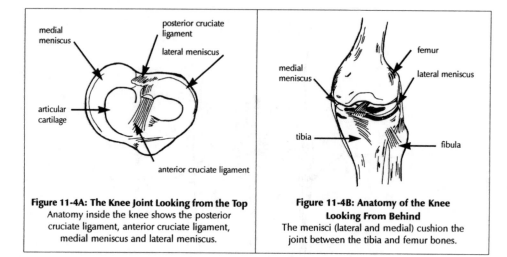

Figure 11-4A: The Knee Joint Looking from the Top
Anatomy inside the knee shows the posterior cruciate ligament, anterior cruciate ligament, medial meniscus and lateral meniscus.

Figure 11-4B: Anatomy of the Knee Looking From Behind
The menisci (lateral and medial) cushion the joint between the tibia and femur bones.

HIP REPLACEMENT SURGERY

In 1994, the National Institute of Health gathered 27 experts in hip replacement and component parts to evaluate hip replacement. In their report, they noted that 120,000 artificial hip joints are implanted annually in the United States. They further stated, "Candidates for elective total hip replacement should have radiographic evidence of joint damage and moderate to severe persistent pain or disability or both that is not substantially relieved by an extended course of nonsurgical management."[10] The National Institute of Health is clearly recommending conservative treatment modalities prior to surgical intervention.

A concern with hip and knee replacements is that the replacement part becomes loose and requires replacement. A loose hip replacement can be treated successfully with Prolotherapy.[11]

KNEE PAIN

It is dangerous to have knee pain and walk into an orthopedic surgeon's office. Apparently, because of the ease of sticking probes into the knee joint, arthroscopic surgery is the favorite pastime of orthopedic surgeons. When I ask patients the reasons for their surgery, the typical response is "to shave cartilage" or "I don't know." The best treatment, as long as it is a partial tear, is to help the body repair the injured area. Remember, removing any tissue that God has put in the body will have a consequence. The tissues most commonly removed during arthroscopic surgery in the knee are parts of the meniscus and the articular cartilage. Both of these structures are needed by the body to help the femur bone glide smoothly over the tibia. **(Figures 11-4)** When either of these structures are removed, the bones do not glide properly. Eventually, whatever meniscus or articular cartilage is left after the arthroscopic surgery is worn away. Once this occurs, bone begins rubbing against bone and proliferative arthritis begins. After a course of cortisone shots, nonsteroidal anti-inflammatory drugs, and several trials of physical therapy, the patient is again under the

the knife, this time for a knee replacement. Once an arthroscope touches the knee, the chance of having arthritis in the knee tremendously increases.

Before letting an arthroscope touch you, it is imperative to have an evaluation by a physician familiar with Prolotherapy. Prolotherapy will begin collagen formation both outside and inside the knee joint depending on the structure(s) that are injected.[12] Prolotherapy stimulates the body to repair itself. Surgery in the knee is appropriate when a ligament is completely torn, such as would occur from a high velocity injury. Prolotherapy is only helpful to regrow ligaments if both ends of the ligament remain attached to bone. Remember, 98 percent of ligament injuries are partial tears for which Prolotherapy would be helpful.

Instability of the knee is effectively treated with Prolotherapy. The following case will illustrate the point. My wife and I received a call from a frantic young woman who was unable to get out of bed because of severe knee pain. We went to her house and found her lying in bed writhing in pain. She explained that as a child she would entertain other children by popping her knees backwards. She had recently seen an orthopedic surgeon to have her knees scraped. He told her that the ligaments in her knees were shot and her only option was knee replacement.

We administered Prolotherapy to her unstable knees. Later that day she was out of bed. In a week, she was back to work. After three sessions she was nearly pain-free. Due to the severity of her case, she received nine Prolotherapy sessions to her knees. That was more than two years ago and she remains pain-free. Prolotherapy strengthens joints. Even in severe cases like this one, as long as the two ends of the ligaments are attached to the bone, Prolotherapy has a good chance of relieving knee joint instability.

DIAGNOSIS OF KNEE CONDITIONS

In diagnosing the cause of knee pain, it is important to carefully examine the knees. A patient whose knees cave inward has a condition known as knocked-knees. **(Figure 11-5)** This stresses and weakens the medial collateral ligament on the inside of the knee. Prolotherapy will strengthen this ligament. Alternately, knees with an outward curvature is a condition known as bow legs. This position applies additional strain on the outside knee ligament, the lateral collateral ligament. **(Figure 11-6)**

It is important to understand the referral patterns of these two ligaments. The medial collateral ligament refers pain down the leg to the big toe and the lateral collateral ligament refers pain to the lateral foot. (*See Figures 2-2.*)

The ligaments inside the knee are called the anterior and posterior cruciate ligaments. These ligaments help stabilize the knee preventing excessive forward and backward movement. If these ligaments are loose, even in a young person, degenerative arthritis begins to form.[13] Prolotherapy causes a stabilization of the knee after these ligaments are treated.[14]

The feeling of a loose knee is reason enough to suspect a cruciate ligament injury. The cruciate ligaments are the power horses that stabilize the knee. They refer pain to the back of the knee. Posterior knee pain may be an indication of cruciate ligament injury.

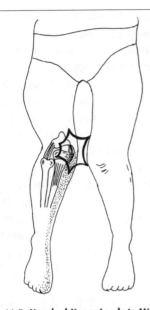

Figure 11-5: Knocked-Knees Leads to Weakness of the Medial Collateral Ligament

Medial collateral ligament weakness refers pain down the inside of the lower leg and foot.

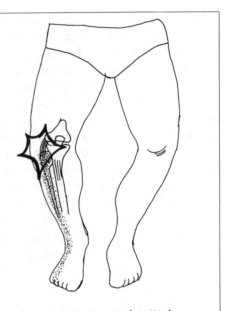

Figure 11-6: Bow Legs Leads to Weakness of the Lateral Collateral Ligament

Lateral collateral ligament refers pain down the outside of the lower leg and foot.

As previously mentioned, the other main structures in the knee are the menisci and the articular cartilage. The menisci consist of a lateral meniscus and a medial meniscus. They are approximately 11 millimeters in length, four millimeters thick, and made primarily of collagen. Prolotherapy injections cause collagen growth. A patient with a meniscus tear should try Prolotherapy before agreeing to see Mr. Arthroscope.

Meniscal injuries are suspected if the patient reports a "catching sensation" in the knee or if the knee must be "jiggled" to produce full range of motion. Articular cartilage injuries exhibit similar symptoms making it difficult to clinically differentiate them. However, they can be differentiated using X-rays.

Prolotherapy is indicated regardless of whether the injury causing the knee pain is due to a meniscal or articular cartilage injury. Prolotherapy injected into a joint requires a more concentrated solution because the joint fluid has a diluting effect. The typical solution for joint injections is 25 percent Dextrose, 20 percent Sarapin, and 0.04 percent lidocaine.

Physicians will traditionally prescribe a nonsteroidal anti-inflammatory medicine like ibuprofen in an attempt to treat an arthritic knee. Arthritis, however, is not the result of an ibuprofen deficiency. The condition producing the arthritis is laxity in some structure of the joint. **(Figure 11-7)** In the knee, the laxity is typically from one of the cruciate or collateral ligaments. When articular cartilage or meniscal tissue is removed from the knee, additional stress is placed on the rest of the knee's

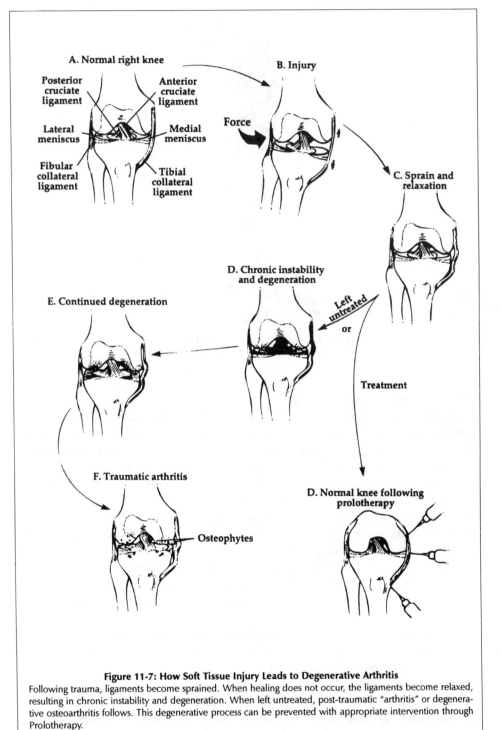

Figure 11-7: How Soft Tissue Injury Leads to Degenerative Arthritis

Following trauma, ligaments become sprained. When healing does not occur, the ligaments become relaxed, resulting in chronic instability and degeneration. When left untreated, post-traumatic "arthritis" or degenerative osteoarthritis follows. This degenerative process can be prevented with appropriate intervention through Prolotherapy.

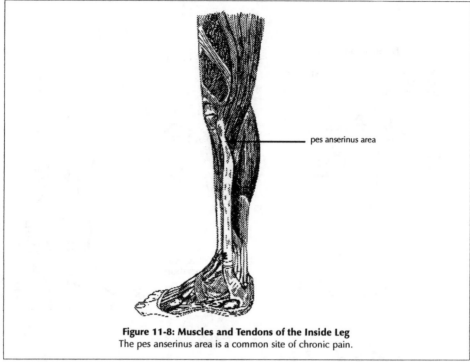

Figure 11-8: Muscles and Tendons of the Inside Leg
The pes anserinus area is a common site of chronic pain.

supporting structures as in arthroscopic knee surgery.

A patient with knee pain will often see Mr. Arthroscope instead of Mr. Prolotherapist, and the result is the articular cartilage on the inside of the knee is removed, as well as some of the medial meniscus, leaving the patient with a reduced amount of cushion on the inside of the knee. Walking now necessitates increased ligamentous support of the knee to maintain stability, eventually causing ligament laxity and pain. This ligament laxity causes the muscles of the pes anserinus and tensor fascia lata to tighten in an attempt to stabilize the knee. The muscles will inevitably break down, resulting in an increase in pain. The tissue on the inside of the knee deteriorates causing additional stress on the ligaments exacerbating the pain. The body, in an attempt to stabilize the joint, grows more bone. This additional growth of bone is called arthritis. Arthritis is the body's attempt to stabilize a joint. The end result is another trip to the orthopedist's office, this time for knee reconstruction.

A much more beneficial approach is to repair the meniscal tissue or any weakened ligament with Prolotherapy. This will prevent the downward spiral of events that lands you in the orthopedist's office.

The most common cause of knee pain is not ligament injury. (I realize that this is shocking, since I have been explaining that ligaments are normally the cause of chronic pain.) The most common cause of chronic knee pain is weakness in the pes anserinus tendons. Below the knee cap, on the inside of the knee, are the attachments of three tendons: semimembranous, semitendinosus, and gracilis. Together, these tendons create the pes anserinus area. **(Figure 11-8)**

I remember coming across a classic pes anserinus case while on rounds as a new doctor in the hospital. A 35-year-old nurse, told me her rheumatologist diagnosed her with arthritis and had prescribed anti-inflammatory medicine. I examined her knee and found that she had full range of motion. Full range of motion of the knee makes it likely that arthritis is not the cause of the knee pain. I took out my reproducibility instrument (my thumb), pressed it into her pes anserinus area and hoopla-bingo! A positive "jump-off-her-chair sign" was elicited. She had pes anserinus tendonitis. I told her about Prolotherapy but she never chose to have treatment. She probably still suffers from the pain, because "arthritis" was not the cause. Even in cases where arthritis is the cause, it is never caused by an anti-inflammatory medication deficiency. Interestingly enough, if someone takes anti-inflammatory medication long enough they will probably get arthritis. Maybe her rheumatologist was talking about the future?

When I give a presentation, I enjoy asking the audience, "What is the number one reason for severe knee pain in the elderly?" The overwhelming response is arthritis, which is incorrect. The number one reason for severe knee pain in the elderly is pes anserinus tendonitis which, when left untreated, may contribute to developing arthritis. Even in cases of significant arthritis, crippling knee pain is most often due to pes anserinus tendonitis or bursitis. This condition is easily treated with Prolotherapy, eliminating the chronic knee pain.

The pes anserinus tendons are also known as the inside hamstring muscles. Most of us have very, very, very weak hamstring muscles that are very short because we sit for a large portion of our day. The pes anserinus tendons flex the knee and stabilize the inside of the knee. Patients with fallen arches are prone to strains in these muscles. The tibia tends to rotate outward to compensate for the fallen arch. **(Figure 11-9)** This outward rotation of the tibia places additional stress on the pes anserinus tendons. Eventually, these tendons become lax and are no longer able to control the tibial movement, adding to the chronic knee pain. An arch support may be prescribed to reestablish the arch. Prolotherapy injections along the arch of the foot will also prove beneficial. Prolotherapy injections into the pes anserinus attachments to the bone strengthen the tendon attachments of the pes anserinus resolving the chronic knee pain. The next chapter will provide more information on ankle and foot pain.

OSGOOD-SCHLATTER DISEASE

Chronic knee pain may develop in young people, especially teenage athletes, and is often due to Osgood-Schlatter Disease, a condition whereby the tibial tubercle becomes painful where the patellar tendon attaches to the tibia. **(Figure 11-10)** Pain occurs because the tendon attaches to the same area of the tibia that is growing. The pain is exacerbated by physical activity, especially running and jumping, and often limits participation in sports, resulting in the young athlete's physician recommending cessation of playing sports. Needless to say, this advice is not popular. A better treatment is to strengthen the fibro-osseous junction of the patellar tendon onto the

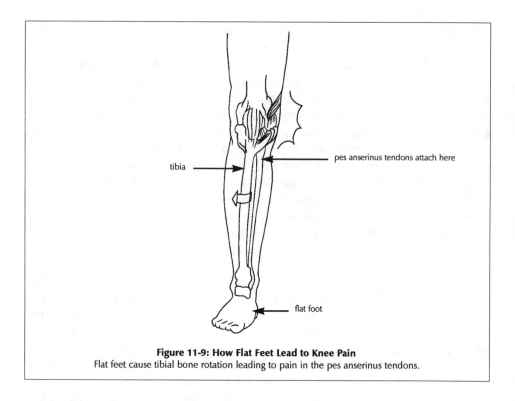

Figure 11-9: How Flat Feet Lead to Knee Pain
Flat feet cause tibial bone rotation leading to pain in the pes anserinus tendons.

tibial tubercle, eliminating the problem.

In a small study published in 1993, Prolotherapy was 83 percent effective in eliminating the pain of Osgood-Schlatter Disease.[15] In this study only one to two treatments were needed to resolve the problem.

CHONDROMALACAE PATELLAE

Another common source of knee pain is known as chondromalacae patellae. (Chondro means cartilage, malacae means breakdown, and patellae means knee cap). Thus chondromalacae patellae refers to cartilage breakdown underneath the patellae. This condition is also called patellofemoral dysfunction or patellar-tracking dysfunction.[16] A more accurate description is that chondromalacae patellae begins as a patellar tracking problem. This means that the knee cap scrapes the bones underneath when the knee is moved. Typical conventional treatments for this condition include taping the knee, exercising to strengthen the thigh muscles, and stretching exercises. These treatments may be effective, but are usually not curative.

Prolotherapy should be considered as a treatment option, especially for resistant cases. If the patella does not track properly in the femoral groove, it may be due to a weakened vastus medialis muscle. The problem would be solved if this muscle could be strengthened independently of the other muscles of the knee. Unfortunately, this is impossible. There is a treatment, however, that can preferentially strengthen one tissue at a time. Do you know what it is? Prolotherapy injections at the site of

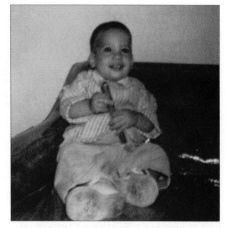

Me at age one. Little did I know that my future included becoming a doctor.

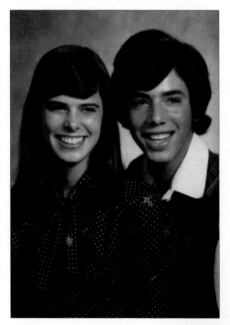

How Marion and I looked when we started dating at 18 years of age.

Marion and me rooting for the Fighting Illini Rosebowl-bound football team while we were students at the University of Illinois.

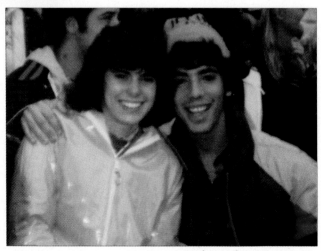

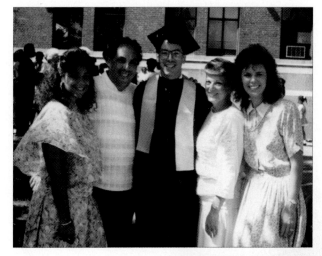

Marion and my family were right there by my side when I graduated from medical school. (From left: my sister Staci, Dad, me, Mom, Marion)

I was happy that my grandparents, Morrie and Eve Groobman, could be there with me on my big day.

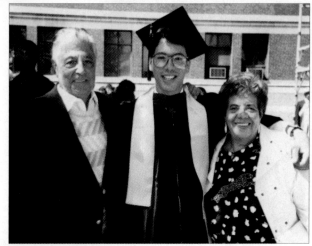

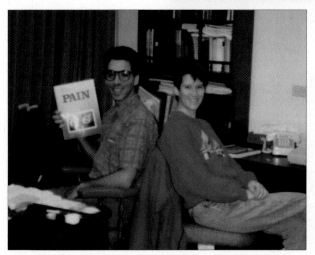

Ross and Elizabeth (my sister-in-law) when Caring Medical and Rehabilitation Services, S.C. was in its early stages. Notice my book on pain.

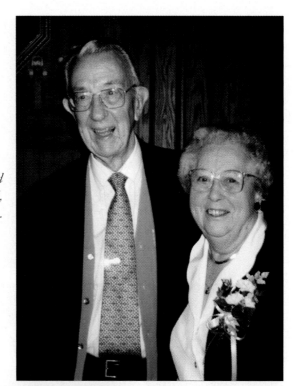

The world's most experienced Prolotherapist, Gustav A. Hemwall, M.D., and his wife, Helen.

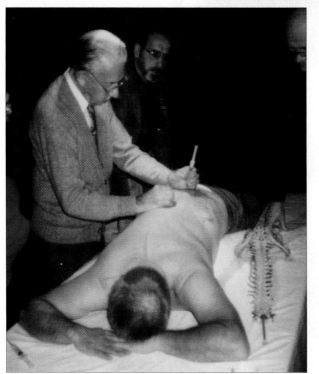

Dr. Hemwall demonstrates using Prolotherapy to alleviate chronic pain to other doctors at the George S. Hackett Prolotherapy meeting in 1992.

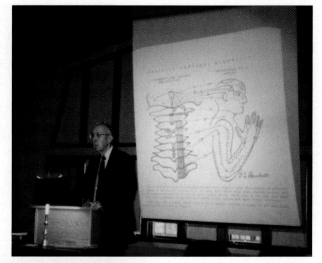

Dr. Hemwall lectures on Prolotherapy at the Hackett foundation meeting in 1992. Notice the Hackett referral pattern of the neck ligaments on the screen behind him.

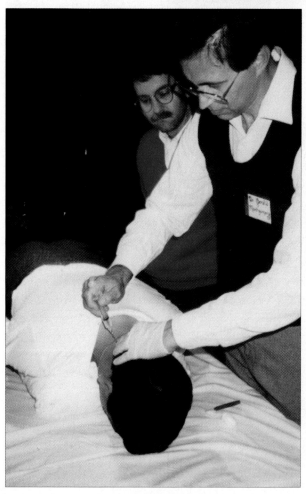

I practice what I preach. Here, I receive Prolotherapy on my neck from Gerald Montgomery, M.D.

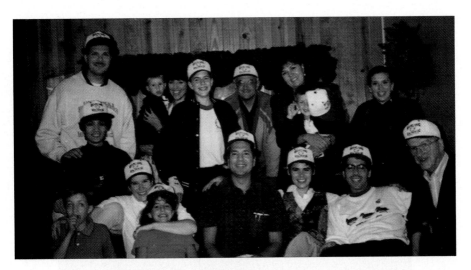

The gang at Beulah Land Natural Medicine Clinic in Thebes, Illinois.

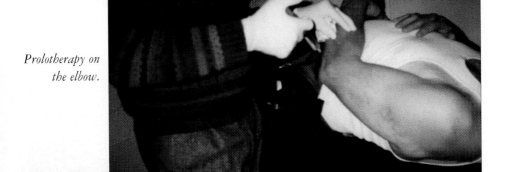

*Prolotherapy on
the elbow.*

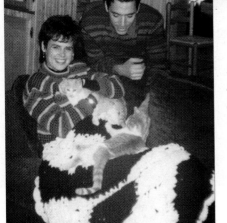

*Marion and I at our house in Thebes with
Squeaky the cat who faked an injury and later
became our permanent companion.*

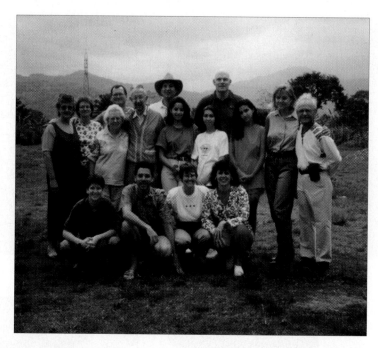

The Prolotherapy crew on a mission trip to Honduras.

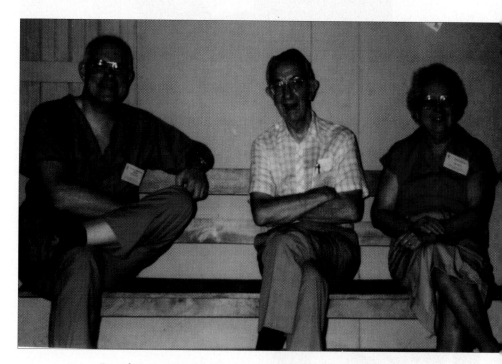

*David Brewer, M.D., Dr. Hemwall and Mrs. Hemwall after the
Prolotherapy clinic during the 1993 Honduras mission trip.*

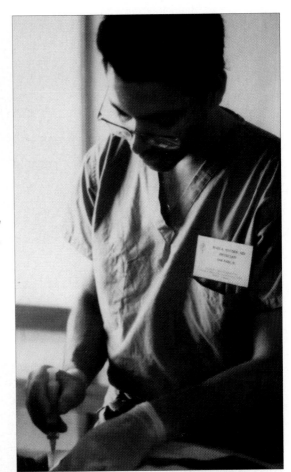

Dr. Hauser doing Prolotherapy in Honduras.

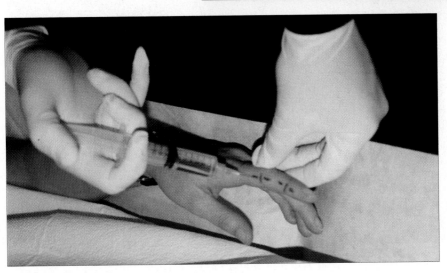

Prolotherapy of the finger.

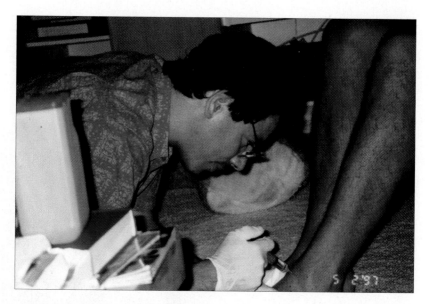

Prolotherapy is such a simple technique that it can be given almost anywhere. Here, I'm visiting a patient in his home and using Prolotherapy to relieve foot pain.

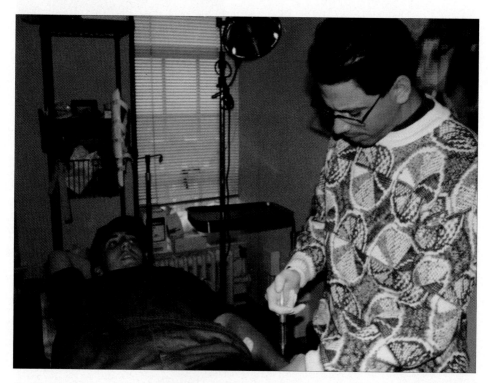

Professional tennis player Gregg Hill flew in from Florida to receive Prolotherapy on his wrist, shoulder and knee. Prolotherapy treatments have enabled Gregg to play tennis pain-free.

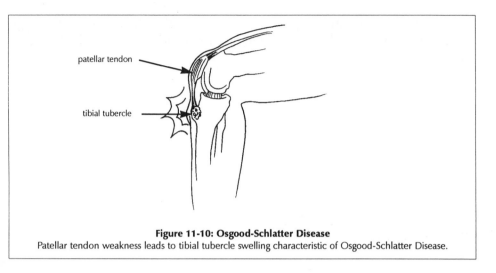

Figure 11-10: Osgood-Schlatter Disease
Patellar tendon weakness leads to tibial tubercle swelling characteristic of Osgood-Schlatter Disease.

the weakened muscle attachments onto the knee cap will help alleviate the problem. Prolotherapy injections for chondromalacae patellae are also given intra-articularly (inside the knee joint). Generally, after four sessions of Prolotherapy the anterior knee pain is resolved.

SUMMARY

In summary, "the ankle bone is connected to the knee bone is connected to the hip bone." Due to the tremendous weight placed on the structures of the lower back and leg during walking, it is important to evaluate the leg and back as a unit. There are many overlooked causes for "sciatica," and chronic groin pain. These include pubic symphysis diathesis, ischiocapsular hip sprain, iliolumbar ligament laxity, sacroiliac laxity, Pyriformis Syndrome, trochanteric bursitis, and iliotibial/tensor fascia lata weakness. Prolotherapy to strengthen the weakness in these tissues helps resolve chronic low back pain, "sciatica," and chronic groin pain.

The most common cause of chronic knee pain is weakness in the pes anserinus tendons, even in the elderly. This is often because a fallen arch in the foot causes rotation of the tibia and stresses the pes anserinus tendons which help support the inside of the knee. Prolotherapy injections to strengthen the tendons help resolve the chronic knee pain. An arch support is also recommended to enhance the chances of permanent healing.

Arthritis of the knee is precipitated by the removal of tissue such as the articular cartilage and menisci during arthroscopic surgery. Prolotherapy to help heal tears in the damaged tissue should be attempted before any arthroscopic procedure.

Anterior knee pain due to chondromalacae patella is primarily due to abnormal tracking of the knee cap on the femur bone during movement. This condition is improved by Prolotherapy injections given intra-articularly and at the fibro-osseous junction. This will strengthen the weakened muscles that cause the tracking problem. Anterior knee pain in young athletes is often due to Osgood-Schlatter Disease.

Prolotherapy is extremely effective in eliminating this condition. Because of these facts, many people are choosing to Prolo their chronic groin, hip, and knee pain away.

CHAPTER 12

Prolo Your Ankle and Foot Pain Away

W hen I watch a boxing match, I am amazed to see the pounding those guys take! What's even more remarkable is that they choose to do it. Even that pounding is minor compared to the pounding feet take every day. The average person takes 3,000 to 10,000 steps per day. The foot's job during the process of walking is to traject the body weight up one inch with each step. If, for example, a woman weighing 125 pounds takes 5,000 steps in a day, her feet have lifted 625,000 pounds during that day. If a 150 pound person walks one mile, 60 tons of force is exerted through the small area that encompasses the ankle and feet. Is it any wonder feet are sore by the end of the day?[1]

FOOT BIOMECHANICS

Poor foot biomechanics may be responsible for a myriad of chronic complaints, including pain in the feet, knees, lower back, and neck.[2] The feet act as a spring, propelling the body forward with each step. If the spring is not working, the propelling force must come from the knees, hip, or lower back. Because these areas are not designed to function in this manner, they eventually deteriorate and the chronic pain cycle begins.

The most important factor in evaluating a person's gait (walking cycle) is to observe the stability of the arch and the ability of the foot to spring the body forward. The most important arch in the foot is the medial arch. **(Figure 12-1)** It is abnormal for the arch to collapse during the gait cycle or while at rest. This collapsing of the arch is known as flat feet, or pes planus. A collapsed arch indicates tissue breakdown. Supporting tissue is no longer able to elevate the inside of the foot. The plantar fascia is the first tissue to be affected. Pain resulting from this weakened tissue is called plantar fasciitis. If the condition continues, a terrible thing will occur. The person will pay a visit to a podiatrist and receive a cortisone shot for the inflamed fascia. Cortisone will eventually weaken the fascia. If the fascia is not strengthened, a painful heel spur will result. Prolotherapy to strengthen the fascia is a superior treatment option.

The next affected structures are the ligaments that support the inside of the foot, especially the calcaneonavicular ligament. (*See Figure 12-3.*) When this ligament is weakened, the arch pain will increase. Eventually, the posterior tibialis tendon in the knee must help support the arch. This tendon eventually weakens, resulting in

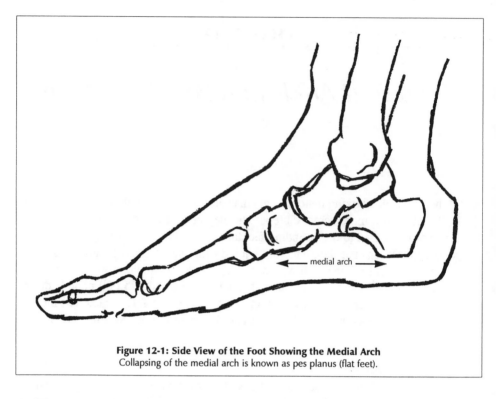

Figure 12-1: Side View of the Foot Showing the Medial Arch
Collapsing of the medial arch is known as pes planus (flat feet).

knee pain added to the original foot pain, as the arch continues to collapse. Because the arch and the knee can no longer elevate the foot, the entire limb must be raised during a step, putting additional strain on the hip. The spring in the foot and the efficiency of the gait are drastically reduced due to the collapsed arch. This requires more energy from the foot, resulting in further deterioration of the medial arch. The more severe the collapse of the arch, the greater the likelihood of pain. The deterioration cycle will continue until something is done to support the arch. Contrary to popular belief, cortisone shots will not accomplish this! Arch pain in the foot is not a cortisone deficiency! **(Figure 12-2)**

FALLEN ARCHES

The medial arch is supported by fascia and ligaments. As previously explained, ligaments maintain proper bone alignment. Loose ligaments allow the bones to shift, resulting in chronic pain. The main supporting structure is the plantar fascia, also known as the plantar aponeurosis. (*Refer to Figure 12-4.*) This plantar fascia is essentially a strong, superficially placed ligament that extends in the middle part of the foot from the calcaneus to the toes. Another important structure is the plantar calcaneonavicular ligament which passes from the lower surface of the calcaneus to the lower surface of the navicular bone. This ligament resists the downward movement of the head of the talus, supporting the highest part of the arch and is responsible for some of the elasticity of the arch. This ligament is also known as the spring ligament.

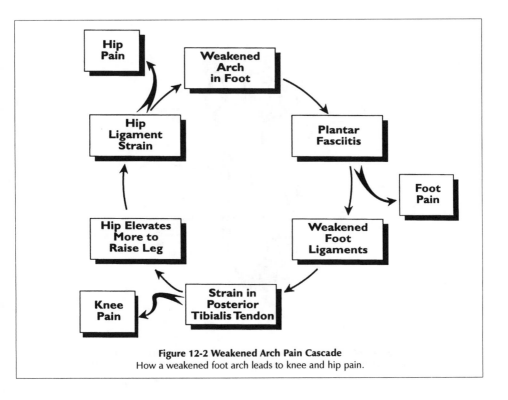

Figure 12-2 Weakened Arch Pain Cascade
How a weakened foot arch leads to knee and hip pain.

An arch support insert is the typical treatment for a fallen arch. Many people experience dramatic pain relief, while others continue to suffer from chronic achy feet. (The only thing worse than chronic achy feet is chronic stinky feet!)

Prolotherapy is the treatment that makes the most sense for a fallen arch due to weak ligaments. Prolotherapy injections into the fibro-osseous junctions of the plantar fascia and calcaneonavicular ligament, which supports the arch, will strengthen this area. If the condition is diagnosed early on, the ligaments can be strengthened to support the arch. If the process has gone on for years, an arch support may be needed in addition to Prolotherapy. But even in the later case, Prolotherapy can eliminate the chronic arch pain.

HEEL SPURS

Many patients with foot pain come to me saying they have been diagnosed with "heel spurs." Others were told they had "plantar fasciitis." Patients have anxiety night and day because they have "heel spurs" and "plantar fasciitis." (It does sound kind of scary, doesn't it?) Such a diagnosis resulted from an X-ray that revealed some extra bone where the plantar fascia attaches to the calcaneus.[3] This extra bone is called a spur. **(Figure 12-4)** Because it involves the heel, it is ingeniously named a "heel spur." It is located where the plantar fascia attaches to the heel, hence plantar fasciitis.

Treatments such as the dreaded cortisone shot or even worse, surgery to remove the spur, have claimed many victims. These treatments do not correct the underlying

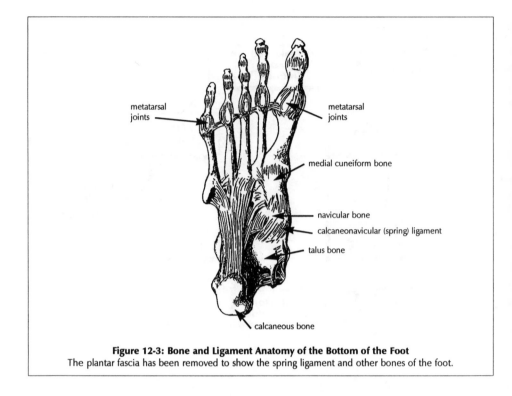

Figure 12-3: Bone and Ligament Anatomy of the Bottom of the Foot
The plantar fascia has been removed to show the spring ligament and other bones of the foot.

defect. The plantar fascia supports the navicular, talus, and medial cuneiform bones. When the plantar fascia must also attempt to support the arch, excess pressure is placed on the calcaneus bone. The calcaneal spur forms because the plantar fascia cannot adequately support the arch. The plantar fascia is "holding on for dear life" to its attachment at the calcaneus. This "holding on for dear life" causes the body to grow more bone in that area in an attempt to reduce the pressure on the ligament, resulting in a heel spur. The same kind of pressure would occur if you were hanging from a ledge of a tall building by the tips of your fingers. You can bet when you were finally rescued that the ledge might have some marks in it where your fingers were located.

Cortisone may temporarily relieve the pain in some cases, but will always weaken tissue long-term. Prolotherapy to the fibro-osseous junction of the plantar fascia will cause a permanent strengthening of that structure. Once the plantar fascia returns to normal strength, the chronic heel pain will be eliminated. "But what about the heel spur?" people complain. Remember, the heel spur is just an X-ray finding. Many people have heel spurs without any pain. Prolotherapy will not remove the heel spur, but it will eliminate the chronic pain by eliminating the cause. So relax and enjoy a foot without pain.

BUNIONS

Bunions are another problem that excite the surgeons. Nothing makes a foot surgeon happier than an elderly patient with bunions. Bunions are an overgrowth of

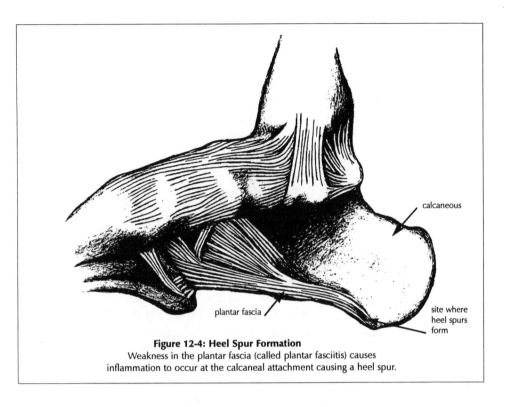

Figure 12-4: Heel Spur Formation
Weakness in the plantar fascia (called plantar fasciitis) causes
inflammation to occur at the calcaneal attachment causing a heel spur.

bone at the first metatarsal phalangeal joint. **(Figure 12-5)** What causes an over-growth of bone? You're learning...ligament weakness. When ligaments weaken, the bones move. This is visually evident because bunions are a result of a gross displacement of the bone. Bone movement due to ligament laxity causes the bones to hit each other. This hitting causes an overgrowth of bone, as an attempt to stabilize the joint. Thus, a bunion is the body's response at the great toe to compensate for a weak ligament.

Prolotherapy eliminates bunion pain. It will not eliminate the toe deformity, but will eliminate the pain. Many people are satisfied with that because don't we all have weird looking toes? You should see my wife's toes, they look like fingers. I believe that if she wanted to, she could eat a meal with her toes. (Please don't try it, honey!)

The foot is similar to the wrist. It consists of several bones in a sea of ligaments. Stretching of any of these ligaments can be a source of chronic pain. John Merriman, M.D., in a 1995 study, obtained good to excellent results in 79 percent of the 204 patients he treated with foot pain utilizing Prolotherapy as the only modality.[4]

ANKLE PAIN

Ankle sprain is likely the most sprained ligament in the body. It is estimated that 26,000 people sprain their ankles every day. Unfortunately, ankle sprains are not always simple injuries and can result in residual symptoms in 30 to 40 percent of patients.[5]

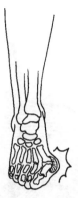

Figure 12-5: Bunion of the Big Toe
Weakness of the ligaments leads to a crooked big toe and subsequent bunion.

The most common ankle sprain is an inversion injury, turning the ankle inward, injuring the ligaments on the lateral side of the ankle, usually the anterior talofibular and the tibiofibular ligaments. **(Figure 12-6)** The most common symptom of this type of injury, besides lateral ankle pain, is a propensity for the ankle to continually turn inward. I suffered from this as a child and it prevented me from ice and roller skating. My ankles would continually turn inward. My ankles were so weak, I did not have the strength to hold myself on skates. Prolotherapy treatments, received as an adult, have eliminated that problem. I still do not ice skate, but that is another issue. Why would any sane person want to be out in the cold, going around and around on a piece of ice?

Exercises designed to strengthen the muscles that support the lateral ankle are beneficial, but rarely solve the problem. Taping ankles, as many trainers and athletes do, only provides temporary benefit. Prolotherapy injections to strengthen the ligaments supporting the lateral ankle provide more definitive results. Chronic ankle sprains are eliminated by Prolotherapy treatments.

The inside of the ankle is held together by a group of ligaments called the deltoid ligament. This ligament is injured from turning the foot outward, as can happen when falling down stairs or mis-stepping. Again, Prolotherapy injections at the fibro-osseous junction of the deltoid ligament eliminate the chronic ankle pain in this area.

MORTON'S NEUROMA & TARSAL TUNNEL SYNDROME
Chronic foot pain and/or numbness

It is quite common for people with the diagnosis of a neuroma, or nerve entrapment, to undergo multiple surgeries attempting to alleviate the entrapment. One individual came to me with a history of 15 surgeries! This occurs primarily because most physicians incorrectly believe numbness is equated with a pinched nerve. Ligament and tendon weakness in the limb also cause chronic numbness in an extremity.

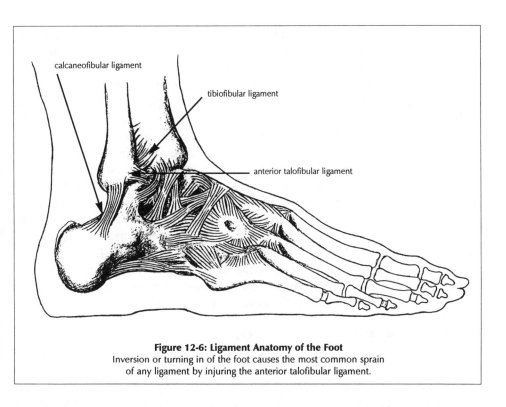

Figure 12-6: Ligament Anatomy of the Foot
Inversion or turning in of the foot causes the most common sprain
of any ligament by injuring the anterior talofibular ligament.

Morton's Neuroma is often diagnosed from the symptom of burning pain in a toe or toes. This is a neuroma involving the nerves located between the toes. These nerves allow sensation to be felt on the skin of the toes. A neuroma is a nervous tissue tumor. Despite years of experimental research and clinical investigation, the painful neuroma has remained difficult to prevent or to treat successfully when it occurs. More than 150 physical and chemical methods for treating neuromas have been utilized including suturing, covering with silicone caps, injecting muscle or bone with chemicals such as alcohol, and many others.[6]

Surgical treatment has been problematic with poor results and complications. In one study, 47 percent of the patients continued to have symptoms of foot pain after surgery.[7] The reason for continued symptoms after surgery or chemical injections may be that the chronic foot pain or numbness is due to ligament weakness and not a pinched nerve.

Tarsal Tunnel Syndrome

Another diagnosis used for chronic burning foot and/or toe pain is Tarsal Tunnel Syndrome. Tarsal Tunnel Syndrome is very similar to Carpal Tunnel Syndrome of the hand (*See Chapter 10.*) except it involves the foot. The tibial nerve runs in a canal on the inside of the foot called the tarsal tunnel. When the tibial nerve gets pinched here, it is called Tarsal Tunnel Syndrome. The symptoms described for this syndrome include pain in the ankle, arch, toes, or heel.[8]

Chronic burning arch, toe, or heel pain is most often due to ligament weakness at the ball of the foot or soft tissue weakness in the arch of the foot, rather than pinching of a nerve as in Tarsal Tunnel Syndrome. The ball of the foot is called the metatarsal joints and supports half the body weight during walking.[9]

Since these structures bear the bulk of the body weight when a person stands, walks, or runs, it is no wonder that these are generally the first structures to weaken. Metatarsal ligament weakness is manifested by pain at the ball of the feet which often radiates into the toes. This is called metatarsalgia. (*See Figure 12-3.*) A weakened arch causes the foot to feel weak and tired especially after a day of standing or walking. It can also radiate pain into the big toe side of the foot. Chronic metatarsal ligament weakness and arch weakness (also known as plantar fasciitis) can cause numbness in the foot and toes in the same areas of pain. Pain and numbness in the foot can also be caused by ligament and tendon laxity in the knee. The lateral collateral ligament can refer pain and numbness down the lateral side of the leg and foot and the medial collateral ligament down the medial side. (*Refer to Figure 11-5 and 11-6.*) Thus anyone with foot pain or numbness needs to have their knees looked at to see if there is any evidence of ligament weakness there.

REFERRAL PAIN PATTERNS OF THE FOOT

As we all know, the foot bone is connected to the leg bone, is connected to the hip bone is connected to the back bone. The hip and back also need to be poked on if someone suffers from foot pain and/or numbness. Hip joint weakness and ligament laxity can refer symptoms to the big toes. The sacroiliac joint commonly refers pain to the lateral foot area. The sacrospinous and sacrotuberous ligaments in the pelvis refer pain and/or numbness to the heel area. So all these areas must be examined to see if they are contributing to a person's symptoms.

It is quite common for a doctor to limit an examination of a patient with foot pain to just the foot. This is a mistake, as foot pain is often a reflection of a knee or back problem. Treatment directed at the foot in such an instance most likely will have unsatisfactory results.

Most chronic foot pain and numbness is not due to a nerve being pinched but due to weakness in the ligaments and soft tissue structures that support the ball of the foot and the arch. Prolotherapy injections start these areas to grow new and stronger tissue. Once this tissue gains normal strength the pain, numbness, and disability stop. If there is evidence for weakness in the ligaments of the knee or back then these are also treated. In Dr. Hemwall's experience treating thousands of patients with chronic foot pain, nerve entrapment surgery was never required. Generally, after four treatments with Prolotherapy the person experienced total resolution of the pain and/or numbness.

Many people, despite surgery, still have pain in their feet from so-called Morton's Neuroma or Tarsal Tunnel Syndrome. The reason for this is that chronic foot, heel, toe, or arch pain is most often due to ligament weakness in the metatarsal joints, or weakness in the plantar fascia that supports the arch. Ligament weakness around the knee, hip, sacroiliac joint, or pelvis can also cause radiating pains and numbness into the foot area. Prolotherapy injections help strengthen these areas. Once they are strong, the chronic foot, heel, arch, and toe pain subsides.

SUMMARY

In summary, chronic ankle and foot pain is relatively common and almost expected, as the feet bear tons of force every day just from the process of walking. Often, chronic foot pain begins from a collapse of the medial arch. This occurs because the spring ligaments and plantar fascia can no longer support the arch. Treatments, such as arch supports, may provide temporary benefit. Prolotherapy injections to strengthen the arch provide permanent results.

"Heel spurs" are due to weakened ligamentous support of the plantar fascia. Prolotherapy to strengthen the plantar fascia will eliminate chronic heel pain. Bunions, an overgrowth of bone, are due to weakness of the metatarsal ligaments. Prolotherapy eliminates the pain of bunions, but does not correct the deformity.

The most common ligament injury is the ankle sprain. Taping and exercising for this condition often have only temporary results. Prolotherapy can permanently strengthen the ligaments of the ankle, eliminating chronic ankle sprains. Because Prolotherapy helps grow the ligaments that are associated with bunions, "heel spurs," "plantar fasciitis," ankle sprains, fallen arches, and Morton's Neuroma, chronic pain from these conditions is eliminated. It is for this reason that many people are choosing to Prolo their chronic ankle and foot pain away.

CHAPTER 13

Prolo Your Fibromyalgia Pain Away

W hen a person first seeks help for pain, a specific diagnosis such as tendonitis is generally given. When the pain continues, an MRI scan or some such study will be ordered. The diagnosis then changes to a "disc problem." After more unsuccessful treatments, the pain sufferer will be sent to a pain center where the diagnosis of depression will be made. After several thousands of dollars of treatment, diagnostic tests, and a lot of frustration and misery, the person will be given that all-inclusive, "so everyone will know I'm not crazy" diagnosis: fibromyalgia. Nearly anyone who has had pain long enough and seeks enough medical opinions will eventually be labeled with this diagnosis.

It is important to remember that nothing of the etiology is revealed when a physician gives a patient a "diagnosis" with the word "syndrome" on the end of it. A "syndrome" is what physicians call a constellation of symptoms for which the actual cause is unknown. A good example of this is what I call the "couch potato syndrome." This syndrome typically describes a balding, middle-aged man with a "basketball-belly" who enjoys watching, talking, and reading about sports, but couldn't walk around the block without getting chest pain. People with this syndrome typically reside in a lounge chair that envelops the body upon contact and a remote channel changer is a must. You see, the physician "diagnosed" "couch potato syndrome," but this says nothing about the etiology of the condition.

It is much more important to know the cause of pain than to have a label placed on it. The diagnosis of fibromyalgia, chronic pain syndrome, or Myofascial Pain Syndrome does not determine the etiology and thus the cure for the condition.

DIAGNOSIS OF FIBROMYALGIA

Traditional medicine will label someone with fibromyalgia if they meet certain diagnostic criteria.[1] Unfortunately, the criteria are somewhat vague. The main criterion is the presence of aches or pains at more than four sites for more than three months with no underlying condition causing the pain. This is why I believe this "diagnosis" is erroneous because a cause for chronic pain can almost always be found. Other symptoms by medical history that cause someone to be labeled with fibromyalgia may include pain in at least 11 of 18 specific tender points, (**Figure 13-1**) a "hurt all over" feeling, anxiety or tension, poor sleep, general fatigue, and/or irritable bowel syndrome.[2]

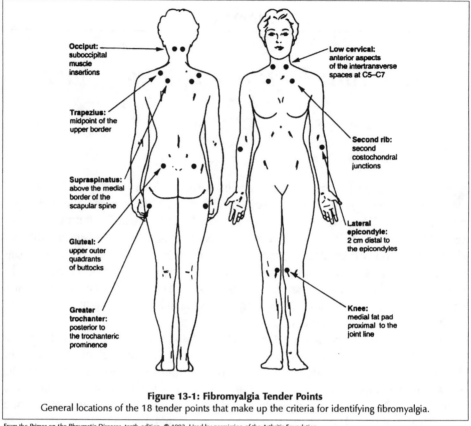

Figure 13-1: Fibromyalgia Tender Points
General locations of the 18 tender points that make up the criteria for identifying fibromyalgia.

From the *Primer on the Rheumatic Diseases*, tenth edition, © 1993. Used by permission of the Arthritis Foundation.

FIBROMYALGIA CASE STUDY

Pamela came to my office with the diagnosis of "fibromyalgia." She told me that about eight years ago, the plague of migraine headaches began. Pamela received several medications for this which provided some relief. She had also been taking antibiotics during this time for chronic sinus infections. After several years, she started having trouble sleeping and felt very tired. She tried chiropractic care, physical therapy, and had seen several orthopedists, neurologists, and internists for what she said was an aching of the muscles. Her X-rays and blood tests were normal. Eventually, she consulted a rheumatologist who diagnosed her with fibromyalgia. She was happy that her condition had finally been diagnosed, but she soon became depressed when she learned that there were no treatment options available and that the current recommendation was that she must "learn to live with it."

My advice to anyone with the diagnosis of "fibromyalgia" is to find a Natural Medicine physician immediately. Only a doctor who practices Natural Medicine will offer any advice that has the potential to be curative for the fibromyalgia patient. Doctors who practice Natural Medicine know that the constellation of symptoms known as "fibromyalgia" can be cured.

The key to Pamela's history was that the condition started in her neck. She noted, after further questioning, that her neck was constantly sore. This was indicative of ligament laxity and was found on palpatory examination eliciting a positive "jump sign." Prolotherapy was performed on her neck. The chronic ligament laxity which led to the neck pain and migraine headaches also caused her to have chronic insomnia. People with chronic pain typically do not get much deep sleep.[3] That is why they wake up feeling nonrested even after 10 hours of sleep.

THE IMPORTANCE OF SLEEP

Upon falling asleep, a person enters stage one and stage two sleep, which is a very light sleep. After approximately 90 minutes, the person will enter stage four, or deep sleep. It is during deep sleep that hormones, like growth hormone, are secreted. Growth hormone, as you will recall, is one of the anabolic hormones that the body needs to repair itself. If a person does not enter the deep stages of sleep, the ability to repair injured tissue is hampered. More than 50 percent of body weight is muscle tissue. It is imperative that the body is able to repair this muscle tissue from its daily use. The body does its repair during the deep stages of sleep. If this is not accomplished, the end result is muscle aching. Do you see the cycle? A person has a localized pain, such as neck pain, that does not resolve. Eventually, the chronic pain causes chronic insomnia. The chronic insomnia causes a decrease in the body's ability to repair itself. This causes pain to move to other parts of the body, causing more insomnia. A vicious cycle continues.

In a 1976 study, Harvey Moldofsky, M.D., solicited healthy volunteers and allowed them to sleep only in stages one and two. Dr. Moldofsky put electrodes on their heads and gave them a little zap, not enough to wake them but enough to keep them from achieving stage four sleep, the deep stage of sleep.[4] Guess how long it took before the previously healthy volunteers had diffuse body aches, tender points, and symptomatology exactly mimicking fibromyalgia? Seven days! In other words, after seven days of nonrestful sleep, these previously healthy people met all the criteria for fibromyalgia, except for the chronicity of the problem.

We all know what this is like. For two days your throat feels scratchy, but you tell yourself, "Nah. I'm not sick." You work another 12-hour day. You mow the lawn, clean out the garage, and do the grocery shopping. The next day you say, "Yeah, I'm sick," as you lay in bed looking for sympathy. After a few days of laying in bed fighting a fever and runny nose, your entire body hurts. It's stiff, sore, and you are exhausted. Do you have fibromyalgia after this? Of course not; you have a cold. Chronic insomnia is the number one reason people have diffuse body aching. To cure diffuse body aching, the cause of the chronic insomnia must be found.

If the chronic insomnia began because of a pain complaint at a particular part of the body, then there is an excellent chance that Prolotherapy can cure the problem. If the chronic insomnia is due to a marital problem, job stress, or other psychological issues, then this is the area that needs to be addressed. Everyone should find a way to reduce their stress level. Let's face it. We all experience stress in our lives.

Realizing that God loves me is my best stress reducer. My slate is clean before Him because I accepted Jesus Christ as my Savior. Jesus took all of my sins upon Himself at the cross when He died. His perfect life is attributed to me before God because I personally accepted Jesus Christ as my Savior. What I have to look forward to is an eternity with God. The Bible says in Revelation 21:4, referring to heaven, "there will be no more pain...." It is hard to be sad and stressed knowing that streets paved with gold are awaiting me. Personal prayer and Bible reading are wonderful ways to keep life's priorities in focus.

There are many other ways to reduce the stress of life. Exercise is the most natural way to reduce stress, as well as help your body attain a deep sleep. We all know what it is like to be totally exhausted from physical labor and sleep "like a baby." We achieved the deep sleep our body was craving.

DEPRESSION

What about depression? Many people with chronic pain are diagnosed with clinical depression as the cause of their chronic pain. My response to this is: Follow the person who made that diagnosis and punch him in the back every five minutes. How long do you think it would be before he or she, too, is depressed? It would probably be similar to the study done by Dr. Moldofsky. After seven days of pain, a previously healthy person can show signs of clinical depression. If a previously healthy person develops chronic pain and is diagnosed with depression, it is logical that chronic pain relief will alleviate the depression. This is exactly what occurs. When Prolotherapy is given to the painful area, the chronic pain dissipates and the smile returns to the patient's face. There have been many sour-faced individuals upon first arrival to my office who later began to enjoy life again. It is amazing what pain relief can do to a person's countenance.

YEAST INFECTIONS

In regard to Pamela, the other clue to her case was that she had been on several antibiotics. Antibiotics destroy the normal and necessary bacteria in the intestine and cause candida (yeast) overgrowth. We tested for yeast antibodies in her blood and found high levels present. How did the yeast get into the blood for her immune system to develop antibodies against it? It came through the intestinal wall. Thus, Pamela's intestinal wall was too permeable (leaky).

Herbs and medicines to kill the yeast were prescribed and she was advised to take acidophilus to replenish the normal bacteria. She was also advised to follow a high protein, low carbohydrate diet—necessary for someone with this condition. (*See Appendix A, Natural Medicine Resources, for information on the nutritional aspects of healing.*)

FIBROMYALGIA HAS A CAUSE

Prolotherapy is not an isolated treatment. The physician must investigate all possible factors which may be involved with a person experiencing diffuse body pain.

What happened to Pamela? I don't know. We discharged her from the practice. I assume she's enjoying her life somewhere. Her pain? That got discharged too.

Most large hospitals have a fibromyalgia support group. How many people must have been diagnosed with fibromyalgia for the hospital to create a support group? People are told they will have recurrent bouts of chronic pain, always feel tired, and are told to live with it. That would drive anyone to a support group! The last line of a fibromyalgia handout from a Chicago hospital reads, "As the wise physician said, 'Once I began to accept that the road was going to be difficult, then it became easier.'" It may be easier for him, but it would be much easier to treat the cause of the chronic pain and alleviate it than attend support groups and live with the pain.

Chronic pain always has a cause. Other etiologies beside ligament laxity for fibromyalgia-type chronic pain include multiple chemical sensitivities[5], hypoadrenocortisolism[6], hypoglycemia, yeast infection, viral infection[7], chronic insomnia, increased intestinal permeability, nutrient deficiencies[8], and poor tissue oxygenation.

To cure the chronic pain, the underlying etiology of the pain must be treated. It is for this reason that people who have the diagnosis of fibromyalgia will be much better served by a physician or health-care professional who utilizes natural treatments that address the above conditions.

To make the diagnosis of fibromyalgia, one of the cardinal features is tenderness over specific points on the body. The diagnosis is made when at least 11 of the 18 points are tender. The unilateral sites are the occiput (insertion of the suboccipital muscles), inter-transverse ligaments C5-C7, trapezius muscle, origin of the supraspinatous muscle, second costochondral junction (ligament), lateral epicondyle (wrist extensor muscle insertions), gluteal area (gluteus maximus muscle), greater trochanter (gluteus medius muscle insertion), and the medial fat pad of the knee (medial collateral ligament). In essence, 14 of the 18 points are located where either a ligament, tendon, or muscle inserts and the remaining four are in the middle of a particular muscle. (*Refer to Figure 13-1.*) Prolotherapy grows ligament, tendon, and muscle tissue where they attach to the bone, thus eliminating trigger points and the pain of fibromyalgia.

Whether a patient has been given the label of fibromyalgia, Myofascial Pain Syndrome, or post-surgical pain syndrome, the hallmark feature typically is very sensitive trigger point areas. The person often feels a knot in the muscle in that area. These areas are called "trigger points" because they trigger a person's pain if compressed and palpated and cause the positive "jump sign." Trigger points also refer pain to a distal site that becomes painful. In a study published in 1994, K. Dean Reeves, M.D., showed that even in people with severe fibromyalgia, Prolotherapy caused a reduction in pain levels and increased functional abilities in more than 75 percent of patients.[9] In 38 percent of the patients, Prolotherapy was the only effective treatment they ever received. An additional 25 percent said that Prolotherapy was much more effective than any previous treatment. The study showed that overall, 90 percent of the severe fibromyalgia patients benefitted from the Prolotherapy injections.

BENIGN CONGENITAL HYPERMOBILITY

An often overlooked but extremely important reason for chronic body pain is benign congenital hypermobility (BCH). Generalized joint hypermobility (loose joints in the entire body) due to ligamentous laxity occurs in about five percent of the population.[10] This may be a genetic problem. The loose ligaments cause the person to have loose joints. Affected individuals over 40 years of age typically have recurrent joint problems and almost universally suffer from chronic pain. The end result of this condition is often diffuse osteoarthritis.[11]

People with benign congenital hypermobility are prone to bone dislocation. Hypermobile joints are exhibited by bending the elbow or knee past the neutral position, touching the floor with the palm while bending at the waist, and touching the thumb to the forearm. In subtler cases, this condition can only be determined by a physical examination—one of the reasons it is not diagnosed by most physicians. Most physicians are not trained how to adequately examine for joint mobility and ligament laxity—another reason why a person with diffuse body pain should be evaluated by a physician familiar with the technique of Prolotherapy.

Prolotherapy is the treatment of choice for benign congenital hypermobility. It is recommended that all hypermobile joints be treated to prevent the formation of arthritis. Patients with chronic pain from diffuse body ligamentous laxity require more than the normal four Prolotherapy sessions. Patients suffering from BCH may also require some Prolotherapy in the future for maintenance purposes.

EHLERS-DANLOS SYNDROME

J.M. exclaimed, "Without Prolotherapy, I would have died 10 years ago!" J.M. has Ehlers-Danlos Syndrome which causes extreme looseness of the joints. It is an inherited condition in which the connective tissue, made up of ligaments, tendons, and muscles, does not form or heal properly.

Conventional medicine does not have a treatment for regenerating connective tissue and is therefore unable to treat Ehlers-Danlos Syndrome. When J.M. finally consulted Gustav A. Hemwall, M.D., the world's most experienced Prolotherapist, she was confined to a wheelchair. Dr. Hemwall treated virtually every joint in her body, since the disease causes all of the joints to become loose. "It was a miracle!" J.M. told me during her follow-up visit in April, 1997. "I can walk, run, and I'm enjoying life." Because of a genetic defect in connective tissue healing, this particular condition requires periodic Prolotherapy treatments to maintain joint stability.

The usual long-term outcome for people with J.M.'s particular type of Ehlers-Danlos Syndrome is a wheelchair-bound shortened life. Aggressive arthritis forms due to the excessively loose joints, and the joints degenerate beyond repair. Fortunately she received Prolotherapy before this occurred.

MYOFASCIAL PAIN SYNDROME

Myofascial Pain Syndrome (MPS) is a common painful muscle disorder caused by taut bands or trigger points in the muscles.[12] Myofascial trigger points are tender areas in muscles causing local and referred muscle pain. Trigger points may cause the tight muscles and tight muscles may cause trigger points.

Myofascial Pain Syndrome and fibromyalgia are often diagnosed in the same patient. Fibromyalgia patients typically have myofascial trigger points over numerous areas of the body. Unfortunately, traditional physical therapy and myofascial therapy on the trigger point areas often do not resolve the problem.

Most people with trigger points obtain pain relief with traditional physical therapy modalities such as massage, ultrasound, and stretching; however, the results diminish during their way home from the therapists' office. Traditional medical doctors who treat people with trigger points will give various kinds of injections into these areas.[13] Again, the patient will leave the doctor's office happy, only to be disappointed when the pain returns.

If, after months of therapy and muscle trigger point injections, the pain has not subsided, most likely the etiological source of the trigger point has not been addressed. Myofascial Pain Syndrome trigger points are in the muscle. However, the etiology of the problem is in the ligament, not the muscle.

Muscles chronically contract to stabilize a joint. This chronic contraction causes the muscles to become overworked and spasmodic. Therefore, chronic knotting or muscle spasm is an indication that the underlying joint is loose, due to underlying ligament and/or joint laxity. When a ligament is lax or weakened the body's next step to stabilize that particular joint is to tighten the muscle. This is why some people have chronic trigger points and are labeled with Myofascial Pain Syndrome. A better diagnosis would be chronic ligament laxity.

Chronic ligament laxity is not affected by muscle trigger point injections, ultrasound, massage, or stretching. Chronic ligament laxity is relieved with Prolotherapy, as Prolotherapy triggers the growth of new ligament tissue. The strengthened ligament holds the joint in place, the muscle relaxes, and the trigger point subsides. It is for this reason that people with Myofascial Pain Syndrome and trigger points are choosing to Prolo their pain away.

SUMMARY

Myofascial Pain and Fibromyalgia Syndromes are often a catch-all diagnoses used to put names to chronic pain conditions. They are syndromes which are a constellation of symptoms for which traditional medicine has yet to determine the cause. All chronic pain has an etiology. The most common reason for chronic pain is chronic ligament laxity. The second most common reason is chronic insomnia. Other causes of diffuse chronic body pain are multiple chemical sensitivities, hypoglycemia, hypothyroidism, hypoadrenocortisolism, viral infection, yeast infection, increased gut permeability, nutrient deficiency, and poor tissue oxygenation. To cure fibromyalgic-type complaints, these conditions must be evaluated and treated. For this reason, it is recommended that the person suffering from diffuse body pain see a Natural Medicine physician. (*See Appendix A, Natural Medicine Resources, for physicians in your area.*)

Benign congenital hypermobility is also characterized by diffuse body pain, but the cause is lax ligaments leading to loose joints. All people who have diffuse body pains have tender points on various parts of their body. The tender points characteristic of fibromyalgia are primarily the areas where ligaments, tendons, and muscles attach to the bone. Prolotherapy causes the ligaments, tendons, and muscles to grow where they attach to the bone. Prolotherapy has been shown to be a benefit to more than 90 percent of people suffering from severe fibromyalgia, benign congenital hypermobility, and Myofascial Pain Syndrome. Prolotherapy is an effective treatment for people suffering from diffuse body pain when tenderness is elicited over muscle, ligament, and tendon attachments to the bone. It is for this reason that many people with these conditions are choosing to Prolo their pain away.

CHAPTER 14

Prolo Your Arthritis Pain Away

I t is important to first note what arthritis is not. It is not a consequence of old age. It is not a Tylenol or Motrin deficiency. It is not the most common reason for chronic disabling pain—no matter what a person's age. Arthritis pain is not a "live with it" condition. There is always a reason for the pain. The most common reason for chronic pain—regardless of age—is ligament laxity. Prolotherapy injections help strengthen weakened ligaments and eliminate chronic pain.

CAUSES OF OSTEOARTHRITIS

Osteoarthritis almost always begins as ligament weakness. (*Refer to Figure 11-7.*) Joints are composed of two bones covered with articular cartilage, allowing the joint to glide, and ligaments holding the two bones together. Healthy articular cartilage and ligaments enable the two bones to glide evenly over one another when the bones move.

If the ligaments become weak, the bones will glide over one another in an uneven manner. One area of the bone will bear additional weight on the articular cartilage when the joint is stressed. This uneven distribution of joint stress creates an even greater strain on the weakened ligament in order to stabilize this joint. Eventually all of the ligaments of the joint become lax. The more lax the ligaments become, the more unstable the joint. This increases the abnormal weight distribution inside the joint. This continued stress within the joint causes articular cartilage breakdown which causes the bones to glide roughly over each other producing a crunching noise when the joint is moved. Grinding or crunching is a warning sign that a cortisone shot awaits you at your conventional doctor's office, unless something is done.

At some point in this process, the body realizes the ligaments can no longer stabilize the joint. Muscles and their respective tendons will then tense in an attempt to stabilize the area on the weakened side of the joint, adding to the person's discomfort. As the muscles and their tendons weaken, which will occur over time, they become more painful and unable to stabilize the joint. They will often "knot" producing painful trigger points. When the muscles and ligaments can no longer stabilize the joint, the bony surfaces rub against each other. In a last attempt to stabilize the joint, additional bone begins accumulating where the bones collide. This bony overgrowth is called Osteoarthritis. Eventually, if the process is not

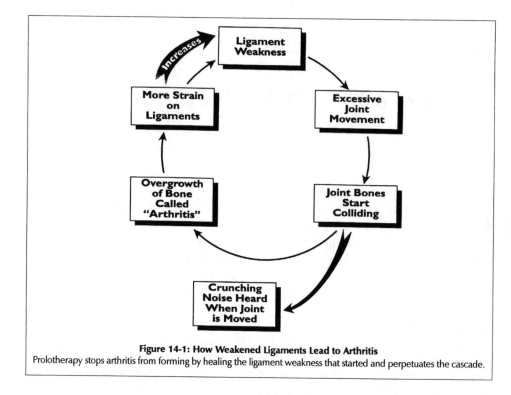

Figure 14-1: How Weakened Ligaments Lead to Arthritis
Prolotherapy stops arthritis from forming by healing the ligament weakness that started and perpetuates the cascade.

stopped at some point, a stiff joint will form.**(Figure 14-1)**

At any time during this process, the body can quickly stabilize the joint by swelling. Swelling of a joint indicates the presence of some foreign substance inside the joint or that the joint is loose. Microorganisms, such as bacteria, blood, pieces of cartilage, and various bodily breakdown products can accumulate in the joints and cause swelling. If a tissue is injured inside and around the joint, typically the joint swells as a protective measure so the body can repair the tissue, which may eventually lead to the development of arthritis.

TREATMENT OF OSTEOARTHRITIS

Acute soft tissue injury, if treated improperly, may begin the cascade resulting in arthritis. As discussed in Chapter Six, icing a joint and taking nonsteroidal anti-inflammatory medicines after an acute soft tissue injury in an attempt to decrease the swelling inhibits the inflammatory mechanisms that heal the body. Treatments such as **R**est, **I**ce, **C**ompression, and **E**levation (RICE) almost guarantee that the joint and the injured tissue will not heal. It is important not to interfere with the body's normal healing mechanism—inflammation—when a soft tissue structure such as a ligament or tendon is injured. Treatment that decreases inflammation after an initial injury will slow and prevent healing resulting in permanently weak tissue, which may eventually lead to the development of arthritis. Treatments that complement the inflammatory process will enhance the healing process.

A better course of action after a soft tissue injury involving a simple sprain of a ligament or strain of a tendon is Movement, Exercise, Analgesics (pain killers), and Treatment (MEAT). It is preferable to use natural botanicals such as bromelain or cayenne pepper as analgesics. In the case of severe pain, a narcotic, such as codeine, works wonderfully to decrease the pain without decreasing the inflammation necessary to heal the tissue. When the body experiences pain, it naturally forms its own narcotic, called endorphins. Completely blocking the pain with narcotics is dangerous because the brain does not recognize that a part of the body is injured. For example, dancing the night away on an injured ankle that feels no pain may cause further damage. Natural botanicals, which do not block all of the pain, are preferred.

Treatment, such as ice, that decreases blood flow to the injured area, causes a decrease in the flow of immune cells, which hinders the healing process. Treatment that increases blood flow, causes an increase in the flow of immune cells to the injured tissue, which triggers the repair process. Movement, exercise, heat, massage, ultrasound, acupuncture, and physical therapy all improve blood flow and have a positive effect on healing.

Attempting to drastically decrease joint swelling after an acute injury is not advisable. The joint swelling is the body saying, "Hey, buddy, I'm hurt. Don't over do it!" Aggressive treatment to decrease the swelling may entice the injured athlete to return to action prematurely. The best course of action is to allow the body to heal itself.

To increase the rate of healing and decrease the length of time the joint is swollen, Protease enzymes are very helpful. Papain and chymopapain from papaya fruit, bromelain from pineapple, and pancreatin enzyme preparations will encourage the removal of the damaged tissue thus reducing the swelling.[1]

An injured ligament not allowed to heal will leave the joint unstable and primed for future arthritis. Prolotherapy blocks the cascade that leads to arthritis by repairing the ligaments that stabilize the joint. The following case study illustrates this scenario.

CASE STUDY

John is a mild mannered accountant who transforms into "Evel Knievel" on the weekend. One weekend while John was skydiving, a gust of wind caused a rough landing. John severely twisted his knee with resultant swelling. His doctor advised him to follow the RICE protocol—Rest, Ice, Compression, and Elevation. John was also given the latest anti-inflammatory medicine, supposedly even stronger than Motrin, called "Strongton."

John's knee pain, a medial collateral ligament sprain, subsided, but the ligament did not heal completely, thanks to the RICE protocol and the anti-inflammatory medicine. Several years later, John noticed occasional grinding in his knee. What John was experiencing was articular cartilage breakdown inside the knee. After several more years, John experienced intermittent pain in the knee. Advertisements persuaded him to take ibuprofen for the pain. Although this relieved the pain, unfortunately for John, the arthritis process was accelerated because his medial collateral ligament injury never healed.

Several years later, John, now in his mid-40s, starts feeling like an old man. In addition to his knee pain, he suffers with a radiating pain down the inside of his lower leg. Not only is skydiving something of the past, but even a simple game of racquetball is a painful experience. John decides to seek medical advice. The doctor X-rays the knee and notices a narrowing of the articular cartilage space. John is told the dreadful news, "John, you have arthritis." At that moment John's mortality flashes before his eyes. The doctor takes out the dreaded prescription pad and writes another prescription for the latest nonsteroidal anti-inflammatory medicine, "Richtin," because it makes the manufacturer rich. What John does not realize is just about everyone who sees that doctor for pain gets exactly the same prescription because that particular drug representative had recently provided the doctor with free samples.

Unfortunately, John does not realize that his pain is not due to a deficiency in any anti-inflammatory medicine. Pain always has a cause, and in most cases the cause can be cured with Prolotherapy. Unfortunately, the physician examined John's knee joint and detected grinding, but did not continue with the necessary palpatory examination. If the physician had been familiar with Prolotherapy and the referral patterns for ligaments, he would have elicited a positive "jump sign" by palpating the medial collateral ligament and pes anserinus tendons. Prolotherapy injections to strengthen the medial collateral ligament and pes anserinus tendons would have stopped the arthritis cascade, as well as eliminate the pain. Once the ligaments and tendons regain normal strength, John would be able to resume his "Evil Kneivel" activities, including sky diving, assuming his ticker was okay and his wife lets him.

Because John's doctor is not familiar with Prolotherapy, the only option John is given is taking anti-inflammatory medicine that is leading him on the road to the orthopedist's office. After several more years, a few more anti-inflammatory prescriptions, and some more X-rays, John's family physician sends him to the orthopedic surgeon, his buddy, "the ortho man."

On the initial visit, John explains that he has medial (inside) knee pain which radiates down the inside of his leg. The orthopedist moves John's knee around and orders an X-ray to assist with the diagnosis. John sweats it out as he waits for the orthopedist to return. "The X-ray shows even further narrowing of the articular cartilage," calmly reports the orthopedist, as a smile begins to form at the corners of his mouth. As the orthopedist gives him the bad news, John's heart races and he feels a lump forming in his throat. "John, your arthritis is worse," says the surgeon. However, John is somewhat relieved, when the orthopedist tells him that he can receive a cortisone shot to help the pain. What John does not realize is his radiating medial knee pain is not due to arthritis. He is also not aware that chronic pain is not due to a cortisone deficiency. The orthopedist proceeds to speed up the arthritis process by injecting John with cortisone into his knee.

At this point, John's lax medial collateral ligament and pes anserinus tendon had still not been addressed. Prolotherapy, even at this juncture, would have halted the arthritis cascade and relieved John's pain.

John's knee feels great for several months after the cortisone shot. He returns as a mad-man to the racquetball court and resumes running again. What John does not realize is the cortisone was masking the pain. His medial collateral ligaments and tendons that support the inside of the knee were getting weaker. The pain relief which allowed John to return to his activities was actually harmful to his condition. His medial collateral ligaments and pes anserinus tendons were not strong enough to stabilize his knee during the racquetball and running. The knee was crying out for him to stop, but was muzzled by the cortisone. Six months later, the pain has returned and John is back in the orthopedist's office receiving another cortisone shot and a new and improved anti-inflammatory medicine.

This process repeats itself several times. John's knee continues to stiffen until one day he realizes that walking is nothing but a painful experience. He limps favoring his bad knee. He sees his buddy the orthopedist. Because they see each other quite often, they have become good friends. The orthopedist recommends another X-ray. Again, John's heart pounds and his hands sweat, as he waits for the report. Soon his stomach feels queasy, like the time he ate that left-over green stuff from the back of the fridge. His heart seems to skip a beat, then his heart leaps into his throat as the verdict is announced. "John, your arthritis has gotten worse." John turns pale, wanting to beg for mercy. His fatal sentence is read, "John, you need a knee replacement." The system claims another victim. Poor John!

John's story is quite common. Perhaps you can relate to it. John's arthritis is severe, but a myriad of natural treatments for arthritis is available. It cannot be overemphasized that chronic disease, whether arthritis, pain, high blood pressure, heart disease, or other disabling conditions, should be managed under the care of a Natural Medicine physician. (*See Appendix C, Natural Medicine Resources, for a list of organizations that supply the names of physicians that utilize natural treatments.*) People generally begin and end with the same treatment system. In the case of chronic pain, if a person starts with traditional medicines like anti-inflammatories, he or she will end up naked in a strange room with lots of funny looking people in masks hovering over him or her. This is called the surgical suite. Anyone who has undergone surgery will agree that it is one scary experience. It is not natural for the body to undergo surgery. In John's case, his pain could have been eliminated with Natural Medicine techniques including Prolotherapy.

Prolotherapy should be instituted and will be beneficial at any point along the arthritis cascade. Prolotherapy will strengthen the supporting structures of the joint, decreasing the pressure on the articular cartilage and the bones of the joint. Prolotherapy will not reverse the arthritic bony changes, but strengthens the joint diminishing the pain. The need for surgical procedures for arthritis can often be eliminated with Prolotherapy.

RHEUMATOID AND INFLAMMATORY ARTHRITIS

Not everyone with arthritis has osteo or degenerative arthritis. Rheumatoid arthritis sufferers make up one percent of the population,[2] another one percent have some other kind of inflammatory arthritis. Inflammatory arthritis generally occurs when the body attacks itself by making antibodies against itself. Antibodies are proteins, made by the immune system, that fight microorganisms such as bacteria that invade the body. In general, people with rheumatoid arthritis manufacture rheumatoid factor, and people with systemic lupus erythematosis produce anti-nuclear antibodies that fight against their own system. In these instances, this inflammation is counterproductive because the body is reacting against its own immune system.

The typical treatment for inflammatory arthritis is anti-inflammatory medicines, often stronger than the usual NSAIDs. Corticosteroids, such as Prednisone, are typically used. As previously stated, chronic pain, no matter the cause, is not due to a medicine deficiency. Rheumatoid arthritis is not due to a Prednisone deficiency. Rheumatoid arthritis does have a cause. Inflammatory arthritis does have a cause. It is for this reason that people suffering from these painful chronic conditions should seek the care of a Natural Medicine physician so the cause of the condition can be treated.

Physicians at the forefront of naturally treating rheumatoid arthritis and inflammatory arthritides are available through contacting The Rheumatoid Disease Foundation. (*See Appendix C, Natural Medicine Resources.*)

CASE STUDY

Physicians who utilize Natural Medicine techniques in the treatment of rheumatologic diseases have all seen cases resolved. Judy, a 34-year-old woman, came to my office complaining of fatigue, body stiffness, and back pain. She was accompanied by her mother who had the obvious hand deformities of rheumatoid arthritis. (**Figure 14-2**) After an initial assessment, I recommended Judy get Prolotherapy injections for the loose ligaments in her back and a blood test for the antibodies associated with rheumatologic diseases. She agreed to both. Oh, if more patients were like Judy. Her blood tests revealed that her body was producing the rheumatoid factor, so I initiated a Natural Medicine program. After six months, her rheumatoid factor was negative. She was pain-free with no signs of rheumatoid arthritis.

NATURAL MEDICINE TREATMENT

Why would the body produce antibodies against itself? Many Natural Medicine practitioners believe the body is trying to fight a microorganism. When the microorganism, such as bacteria, invades the body, the immune system immediately begins making "torpedoes to kill the enemy." The torpedoes that the white blood cells make are called antibodies. In some individuals, the body forms antibodies against the organism and itself. In this case, antibiotic therapy or another treatment to kill the microorganism should cause a relief in the rheumatoid arthritis symptoms, correct? This is precisely what occurs in many individuals.

Natural Medicine clinicians have long suspected a bacterial etiology for rheumatoid arthritis.[3] A recent double-blind study reported the beneficial effects of antibiotics, such as minocycline, for rheumatoid arthritis.[4] Natural antibiotics, such as garlic, goldenseal, echinacea, and grapeseed extract are used by some to avoid the side

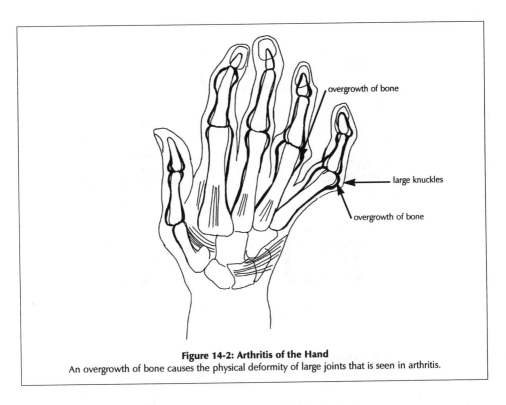

Figure 14-2: Arthritis of the Hand
An overgrowth of bone causes the physical deformity of large joints that is seen in arthritis.

effects of synthetic antibiotics. Many Natural Medicine physicians utilize bio-oxidative medicine techniques, including hydrogen peroxide or ozone therapy, and ultraviolet blood irradiation (Photoluminescence), as anti-microbial therapies. Dr. Hemwall and I use a combination of a bacterial vaccine and influenza vaccine to successfully treat inflammatory arthritis. This vaccine protocol was developed by Bernard Bellew, M.D., who successfully treated hundreds of patients with degenerative and rheumatoid arthritis claiming 80 to 90 percent success rate.[5] The vaccine helps the body fight and kill the microorganism that is causing the arthritis. He has kept patients' inflammatory arthritis, including rheumatoid arthritis, under control for decades by utilizing this Bellew arthritis vaccine protocol.

POSSIBLE CAUSES OF RHEUMATOID AND INFLAMMATORY ARTHRITIS
Intestinal Permeability
Intestinal permeability allows microorganisms and other foreign substances to circulate throughout the body.[6] The "stuff" inside the intestines is actually outside of the body. Contrary to popular belief, you are not what you eat. You are what you absorb. Technically, until something is absorbed it is not inside the body. One of the functions of the lining of the stomach and intestines is to keep out the bad "stuff." Chemicals, heavy metals, and microorganisms are examples of the harmful "stuff." An increase in the intestinal permeability (leaky gut) allows various substances designed to remain in the intestines to leak into the body. **(Figure 14-3)**

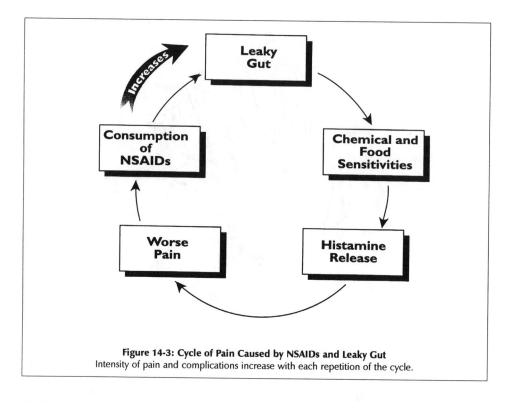

Figure 14-3: Cycle of Pain Caused by NSAIDs and Leaky Gut
Intensity of pain and complications increase with each repetition of the cycle.

Antibodies are then produced as the body attempts to eliminate these toxins. In some individuals these antibodies attack the joints causing rheumatoid arthritis or other inflammatory arthritides. Various chemical and food sensitivities form due to chemicals and food breakdown products leaking into the body. Repeated exposure to these chemicals and foods causes the body to identify them as foreign invaders, releasing histamine and firing antibodies, in response. The histamine and antibody release causes increased intestinal permeability, thereby worsening the arthritis and pain. This vicious cycle will continue until all factors associated with the "leaky gut" are eliminated.

What causes the intestinal permeability in the first place? Heavy metals, medications, infections, allergens, chemicals, tumors, and surgery are often the culprits.[7,8] It is interesting to note the medications Prednisone and ibuprofen are well known irritants and destroyers of the coating of the intestines.[9,10] NSAIDs, commonly prescribed for pain, are some of the worst offenders that cause leaky gut. A bleeding ulcer, the ultimate in increased intestinal permeability, is often the result of taking these medications. This is another reason to avoid these medicines. Rheumatologic diseases are not a Prednisone or anti-inflammatory medicine deficiency. These medications, besides not correcting the problem, may exacerbate the condition.

Poor Diet

Most Americans have very poor diets, consisting of large amounts of highly processed fast-foods that are very low in nutritional value. Many of my patients report that they consume NO fruits or vegetables at all. Typical Natural Medicine treatments for rheumatologic conditions include a very healthy diet that is preservative and chemical free. A diet loaded with organic fruits and vegetables is recommended. An easy way to obtain relief from rheumatoid arthritis is a prolonged juice fast. It is not advisable to attempt any treatment in this book unless under the care of a physician familiar with these techniques. Fasting produces near immediate results because the toxic chemicals and foods are removed and the intestinal lining has an opportunity to repair itself. Every day people subject their bodies to a myriad of chemicals and preservatives from the food they eat. The average American consumes 140 pounds of sugar per year.[11] Is it any wonder that little leaks occur in the system with this kind of assault on the stomach and intestine? A healthy diet free of pesticides, chemicals, and preservatives is necessary for good health. It is, of course, vital to healing the body of rheumatoid arthritis. (*See Appendix A, Nutrition and Chronic Pain for more information on nutrition.*)

Heavy Metals

As previously mentioned, the intestinal permeability is also increased by heavy metal exposure. Patients ask me, "how did I get heavy metals?" Open your mouth and take a peek. Amalgam fillings contain a plethora of heavy metals. They are typically comprised of 50 percent mercury, and the rest various alloys of silver, tin, and nickel.[12] Gold fillings, in actuality, contain very little gold, but are made up of various alloys of silver, tin, and nickel. Since saliva is often acidic, guess what happens when heavy metal is placed in this acid environment? The metals solubilize, meaning the mercury, silver, and tin bond with the saliva which travels to the stomach and wreak havoc on the digestive tract. One of the results is leaky gut syndrome or intestinal permeability. Natural Medicine physicians typically check the hair, urine, and blood for heavy metals in people with chronic conditions like rheumatoid arthritis. An amazing amount of waste accumulates in a person's body over the years such as mercury, silver, and tin. It is highly advisable to remove these as they have a detrimental health effect.[13] A course of chelation therapy is often recommended to remove the heavy metals from the body. (*See Appendix C, Natural Medicine Resources, for resources on chelation and Natural Medicine physicians.*) Removal of amalgam fillings is sometimes advised for patients with accumulation of heavy metals.

Another result of heavy metal in the mouth is the formation of a battery. Acidic saliva combining with metal in the fillings produces the "battery." I do not know about you, but I do not want a battery only two inches from the base of my brain. Amalgam fillings should be removed by a biological dentist (mercury-free) to prevent these reactions from taking place in the body.

Omega-3 Fatty Acid Deficiency

It is difficult to imagine with all the hype to lower the fat in our diets that anyone could be fat or fatty acid deficient. You may find it hard to believe, but some fat is good. Most Americans unfortunately have too much fat that hangs over their belt lines due to the over consumption of total calories. Another type of fat that causes trouble are Omega-6 fatty acids. These fatty acids are increased in the body because of consuming too many foods fried in hydrogenated vegetable oil and the consumption of other hydrogenated oils such as those found in margarine. Hydrogenated oils are everywhere! Look at the labels the next time you purchase crackers, cookies, and salad dressings. You will be surprised to find that almost all baked goods contain them.

Over consumption of fried foods, margarine, and other foods with hydrogenated oils will increase the body's inflammatory state and make the symptoms of disease such as rheumatoid arthritis worse. The way to counteract this is to stop porking out on pork fritters and start eating salmon!

Salmon and other fish contain a high amount of Omega-3 fatty acids. Omega-3 fatty acids have been shown to reduce the incidence of rheumatologic diseases, as well as the symptomatology.[14] The fatty acids in the fish oil, specifically eicosapentaenoic acid (EPA) and docosahexaenoic acid (DHA), dramatically improve the functional ability and diminish the pain in a myriad of diseases, including psoriasis, psoriatic arthritis, gout, lupus, osteoarthritis, and rheumatoid arthritis.[15]

Apparently for optimum health, a ratio of 1:1 in the diet of Omega-6 to Omega-3 is the healthiest. Currently, that ratio in the standard American diet is close to 20:1.[16] Supplementation with such things as flax seed oil, evening primrose oil, borage oil, and fish oils may help bring the Omega-6 to Omega-3 ratio into proper proportion and more toward optimal health. This is why part of standard Natural Medicine treatment for inflammatory arthritis, including rheumatoid arthritis, is the high dose consumption of fish and fish oils. Lipase enzymes are also given so that the fat is digested properly.

Immune Dysfunction

An impairment in the immune system is always associated with chronic disease. This impairment in the immune system will retard soft tissue healing. Someone with a chronic disease, such as rheumatoid arthritis, is more likely to have chronic ligament and tendon laxities due to the deficiency in soft tissue healing. Prolotherapy starts the growth of ligament and tendon tissue, regardless of the etiological cause of the weakness. However, the body actually grows the ligament tissue. The stronger and healthier a person's immune system, the greater the growth of ligament and tendon tissue.

Anti-Inflammatory Agents

Any treatment that decreases the inflammatory response will ultimately slow and potentially stop soft tissue healing and worsen the arthritic condition. Prolotherapy injections cause inflammation which initiates ligament and tendon growth. I recommend avoidance of ice and anti-inflammatory medicines during Prolotherapy treatments. Ice and anti-inflammatory medicines such as aspirin, Motrin, ibuprofen, and Prednisone decrease the healing and growth of tissue that occurs with Prolotherapy.

I have had patients who have needed anti-inflammatory drugs, such as Prednisone, because of another chronic disease, such as rheumatoid arthritis, receive Prolotherapy with good results. This is not the ideal situation however. Weaning the person off the anti-inflammatory medicines prior to starting Prolotherapy is often necessary. Anything that decreases inflammation has the potential to interfere with the healing that occurs with Prolotherapy. Conversely, anything that improves blood flow or strengthens the immune system, has the potential to assist the healing from Prolotherapy. Acupuncture, heat, massage, myofascial release, exercise, electrical stimulation, and physical therapy all improve blood flow and benefit the patient undergoing Prolotherapy.

A person with a chronic disease will often need more than the four sessions of Prolotherapy to heal the ligament and tendon weakness. They often require supplemental therapies to resolve the chronic pain complaint. A patient with chronic pain from inflammatory arthritis caused by tendon or ligament laxity will benefit from Prolotherapy injections. If, however, the joint is hot, red, and swollen, then the pain is likely due to the body's production of antibodies against itself. In this case, Prolotherapy injections to that joint would cause additional inflammation, and intensify the problem. If the pain is due to a loose joint that is not hot and red, then ligament laxity is the likely culprit. In this case, the physician should take out his strong thumb and elicit a positive "jump sign." If elicited, Prolotherapy injections should begin.

SUMMARY

The two main categories of arthritis are degenerative arthritis, also known as osteoarthritis, and inflammatory arthritis, typically rheumatoid arthritis. Ligament laxity is normally the cause of osteo or degenerative arthritis. The weak ligament, if not repaired by Prolotherapy, will eventually lead to a loose joint. The muscles and tendons tighten in an attempt to stabilize the joint. When this fails, the articular cartilage deteriorates on one side of the joint. The bones begin rubbing on that side of the joint. This causes an overgrowth of bone called osteoarthritis. Prolotherapy injections to strengthen the joint stop this arthritis cascade. If osteoarthritis has already formed, Prolotherapy will relieve the pain but cannot reverse the bony overgrowth that has already occurred.

Increased intestinal permeability is one etiology for rheumatoid arthritis and inflammatory arthritis. This increased intestinal permeability causes substances such as chemicals, heavy metals, and microorganisms to enter the body. To eliminate the pain from rheumatoid arthritis, a Natural Medicine approach including a proper diet, avoidance of anti-inflammatory agents, treatment of microorganism invasion, elimination of heavy metals, and a proper balance of Omega-6 to Omega-3 fatty acids is recommended during Prolotherapy.

Typically, Natural Medicine therapies, in addition to Prolotherapy, are necessary to relieve the chronic pain for the chronic disease patient. Prolotherapy is an excellent adjunct to the management of chronic pain from arthritis. Because of these facts, many people with arthritis are choosing to Prolo their arthritis pain away.

CHAPTER 15

Prolo Your RSD, SCI, and Other Neurological Pains Away

P ossibly the worst pain syndrome is Reflex Sympathetic Dystrophy, referred to as RSD. RSD is the granddaddy of pain syndromes. People suffering from RSD experience continual pain that feels like their skin is on fire. To an RSD patient, touching a piece of tissue paper or a bed sheet with the affected limb feels like touching fire.

RSD may appear at any age and is nondiscriminatory, affecting young, old, male, and female. It spreads like wild fire. It may start in the foot, move its way up to the knee, in the back, down the other leg, and up into the arms. People with RSD are panicked, anxious, and searching for anything that will alleviate the pain.

In 1986, the International Association for the Study of Pain Subcommittee on Taxonomy defined Reflex Sympathetic Dystrophy as continuous pain in an extremity with sympathetic hyperactivity. This generally occurs from a trauma such as a bone fracture.[1] The name of the condition was later changed to Sympathetically-Mediated Regional Pain Syndrome. It is a pain syndrome that occurs due to an increase in the activity of the sympathetic nervous system. RSD is very similar to fibromyalgia, in that many people are labeled with both of these conditions when, in fact, they have ligament or tendon laxity. Ligament laxity can cause severe burning extremity pain. Just as with fibromyalgia, traditional treatments usually provide only temporary benefits.

STAGES OF RSD

RSD is a deteriorating disease, progressing in three stages. In stage I, the acute phase, the pain is described as burning or aching which is exacerbated by touch, emotional upset, or active/passive movement. The pain is often tremendous, much more than is expected with the original injury.[2] Two months after a stubbed toe, severe pain may develop far beyond what would normally be expected for such a mild injury. The involved limb becomes edematous (filled with fluid) and may be hot or cold. A bone scan may reveal an increased uptake of the radioactive phosphate compound in the affected area, indicating increased uptake of red blood cells to the area.

In stage II, the dystrophic phase of RSD, the pain is constant and is exacerbated by any sensory input. Excruciating pain is elicited by touching, vibrating, moving, or even blowing on the affected limb. The limb becomes more edematous, cool, and hyperhidrotic (sweaty). The bone scan typically shows a decreased uptake of red blood cells and X-ray films reveal the initial stages of osteoporosis.

Finally, in stage III, the atrophic phase, irreversible damage occurs to the extremity. Because of limited movement of the extremity, the affected limb contracts and the skin becomes cool, thin, and shiny. Because of scar tissue, it is nearly impossible to move the joint and arthritis and osteoporosis are prevalent resulting in a permanently frozen or contracted limb. At this time, the pain begins to subside; however, the limb is now essentially useless. The progression from stage I to stage III occurs over several months or years. Unfortunately, this process may repeat itself in other parts of the body.

CAUSES OF RSD

Factors that predispose people to RSD are arthritis, brain injury, spinal cord injury, fracture, herpes, immobilization with a cast or splint, infection, heart attack, soft-tissue injury, surgery, nerve injury, sprain, tendonitis or bursitis, vasculitis, and others.[3] RSD experts conclude that trauma is the usual initiating event in the development of RSD.[4,5,6]

People experiencing chronic pain attempt to decrease inflammation, most often by taking anti-inflammatory medicines, thereby unknowingly diminishing the chance of healing. The majority of people with RSD have also taken anti-inflammatory medicines after their injury thereby diminishing their chances of healing. In every case of RSD I have treated, the patient was previously advised to immobilize the limb, generally the foot or hand, for a prolonged period of time. Immobilizing an injured joint for a prolonged period of time will guarantee inadequate healing of the soft tissue injury.

The traditional treatment for soft tissue or bony injuries, as previously discussed, is Rest, Ice, Compression, and Elevation. Rest has the following detrimental effects on the bones and soft tissues of the joints after two weeks of immobilization: fibrosis of periarticular tissue (contracture and weakening of joint capsules and ligaments), cartilage deterioration producing an overgrowth of bone, atrophy in weight-bearing areas, and regional bony eburnation, sclerosis and resorption (fancy terms for arthritis and osteoporosis). Many of these effects are irreversible.[7]

Periodic short-term immobilization of the joint also has cumulative harmful effects.[8] Periodic immobilization over 30 days or longer leads to progressive osteoarthritis and will decrease range of motion. An immobilization period of as little as four days has a cumulative effect of producing osteoarthritis. An interval of four weeks between immobilization periods does not prevent osteoarthritis from developing.[9] Think about what this is saying. Only four days of joint immobilization will induce changes indicative of osteoarthritis. A cast on an arm or leg for six to eight weeks or an ankle strap to rest the ankle for a week or two is a lot longer than four days. Remember, we are talking about cumulative days. It is not uncommon for RSD patients to relay a treatment course of resting the limb for a few days, a doctor wrapping it for a week or two, and another doctor casting it for a month. The patient eventually immobilizes the limb because of the severity of the pain. The immobility triggers the arthritic process and potentially the RSD process as well.

Immobility is especially detrimental to the articular cartilage that lines the bones in the joints. The articular cartilage has no blood vessel supply. It depends on the compressive force of the bones to provide joint fluid into the articular cartilage for nourishment. An immobilized joint starves the articular cartilage. Immobility causes a reduction in the cartilage water content, a decrease in the glycosaminoglycan content, and a loss of hexamines from the periarticular tissue.[10] In other words, the articular cartilage degenerates, beginning a slow death of the cartilage. **(Figure 15-1)**

It is common medical knowledge that immobility causes osteoporosis or weakening of the bones,[11] due to the urinary excretion of calcium from the resorption of bone. This osteoporosis process begins as soon as the limb becomes immobile. The strength of the bones is dependent upon muscle contraction through production of an electrical current with each contraction. The greater the immobility the greater the osteoporosis.[12] When a tissue is injured, anti-inflammatories and immobility should be avoided. Movement, Exercise, Analgesics, and Treatment (MEAT) as opposed to RICE, after an injury in many cases will prevent the onslaught of RSD.

It is not uncommon after a cast is removed for pain in the limb to remain. The orthopedist interprets this as a normal occurrence caused by stiffness and recommends physical therapy to resolve the problem. Unfortunately for many, therapy does not resolve the problem; consequently, the patient sees another physician. Many do not find relief, and although they may not develop RSD, they have a chronic pain problem. The solution to their problem may be found with a physician familiar with Prolotherapy.

Imagine the magnitude of force required to break a bone. What happens to the ligaments that support the joint around the broken bone? The ligaments are injured. The blood supply to bone is excellent, whereas blood supply to ligament tissue is poor. Small feeder blood vessels which are sheared during the initial injury are designed to supply the ligaments with essential nutrients. This worsens the nutritional support that the ligaments receive. Combine this with NSAIDs and immobility, and the ligaments have essentially no hope of healing. This is why patients have chronic pain after their cast is removed despite good physical therapy. Post-casting, post-broken bone pain that does not respond to physical therapy is most likely a ligament injury. Weakened ligaments will not heal with physical therapy. Chronic ligament laxity has only one curative treatment, Prolotherapy.

RSD is often triggered by a traumatic event. This initial injury causes soft tissue damage involving the ligaments. The sympathetic nervous system shuts down to allow increased blood flow to the area in order to heal the injury. This is why initial bone scans clearly reveal RSD. Because the ligaments do not heal, joint deterioration continues. As the joint continues to deteriorate, the sympathetic system's output increases because the ligament injury has not healed.

PHYSIOLOGICAL CHANGES OCCURRING IN RSD

What is the source of RSD pain? As the name implies, the sympathetic system becomes hyperactive. The sympathetic nervous system, the adrenaline system, is activated when you are nervous. What causes and maintains the hyperactivity of the

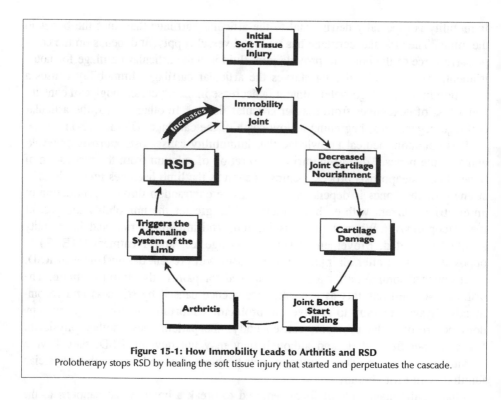

Figure 15-1: How Immobility Leads to Arthritis and RSD
Prolotherapy stops RSD by healing the soft tissue injury that started and perpetuates the cascade.

sympathetic nervous system? The sympathetic nervous system is part of the autonomic nervous system, meaning that it is not under our conscious control. We do not consciously direct our blood vessels to dilate from 1.2 mm in diameter to 1.3 mm because it is a hot day. This happens automatically. For example, it is the bottom of the ninth, your team is down by a run, two outs and bases are loaded and it is your turn to bat. You feel your hands get cold and sweaty, your heart pounds, your blood pressure rises, and if you are a Chicago Cub, you strike out. Sorry, Cub fans!

The sympathetic stimulation on the blood vessels causes them to constrict, therefore, decreasing the blood supply to the tendons, ligaments, bones, and skin of the limb. Decreased blood supply will also decrease the immune system's ability to heal and lead to osteoporosis, and the tendons and ligaments become fibrosed or shortened. The skin becomes shiny and pale. Because of impaired joint movement, the articular joint degenerates. The end result of the increased sympathetic activity is a contracted useless limb. It is imperative to properly treat RSD at the onset of its symptomatology.

In 1949, I. Korr, M.D., published the first of a series of papers on sympathetic hyperactivity related to alterations in the sensory input from the musculoskeletal system.[13,14,15,16] He described how muscle, joint, or soft tissue injury caused an increase in the activity of the sympathetic nervous system at the injured limb. Bio-mechanical stress such as tilting the pelvis or wearing a heel lift could cause the hyperactivity. Other studies have shown that any type of noxious mechanical deformation or chemical irritation of the soft tissues or joints alters the sensory input to the sympathetic nervous system.[17] This causes the sympathetic nervous system to fire the nerves and the blood vessels to constrict in the limb, triggering the progression of RSD.

TREATMENT OF RSD

The traditional treatment for RSD involves various forms of sympathetic nerve blocks, consisting of injections of anesthetics into the sympathetic ganglion in the neck and back.[18,19] These sympathetic ganglion blocks cause an immediate increase in temperature to the limb due to the increased blood flow. Often the patient experiences immediate pain relief.

Unfortunately, this treatment is only temporarily effective. RSD patients may receive multiple sympathetic blocks, to the point of having anesthetic pumps placed in their backs, or even have the sympathetic nerves severed in an attempt to find relief from their pain.

Treating the ligament injuries to stabilize the joint during stage I and stage II will eliminate the symptoms of RSD. An evaluation by a physician familiar with Prolotherapy is crucial for proper diagnosis and treatment for anyone who has had a simple injury that has not healed after several months. Prolotherapy injections to repair injured ligaments will keep a simple injury, simple. The further the progression of RSD, the harder it is to treat. If Prolotherapy is performed prior to the stage III changes, the condition is reversible. Prolotherapy can halt the progression of RSD because the initial etiological basis for the disease, ligament injury, is corrected. For example, RSD of the feet is often due to an injury to the anterior talofibular and its accompanying ligaments.

In prolonged cases of RSD, complementary treatments, which improve blood flow, may be necessary in addition to the Prolotherapy. A complementary treatment for the pain of RSD, which also improves blood flow, is topical application of dimethyl sulfoxide or DMSO. This liquid is applied, typically twice per day, to the skin of the painful limb and has been shown to be very effective in the treatment of RSD pain.[20] Other treatments include chelation therapy, bio-oxidative techniques, heat, exercise, and physical therapy.

Prolotherapy stimulates the body to improve blood flow because it causes inflammation at the fibro-osseous junction. Prolotherapy cannot reverse the destructive changes that have occurred, but can be very helpful in eliminating the pain from RSD.

CASE STUDY OF RSD PATIENT

My patient, Mrs. D., is a typical RSD case. She was in excellent health until she sprained her ankle. After a few days of doctoring it herself, she visited her internist who prescribed NSAIDs. Her pain persisted despite faithful compliance with the prescription. She saw her internist a few more times who prescribed a different NSAID and physical therapy. The next step was a podiatrist who taped the ankle for additional support. Because there was still no pain relief from the ankle sprain, she was fitted for a walking cast to "calm the pain and help the healing." After a month, when the cast was removed, Mrs. D. was left with a stiff sore foot, in addition to her ankle pain. She sought help from several other physicians, and was eventually given the diagnosis of RSD.

When she came to my office, she needed assistance to walk. Pressure readings, taken with a dolimeter, a device that quantitatively measures the amount of pressure necessary to elicit pain, revealed sensitivity to palpation over the entire foot, a hallmark feature of RSD.

I treated her with Prolotherapy to strengthen the ligaments and prescribed topical DMSO to decrease the sensitivity on the foot. She progressed gradually and after four months all pain symptoms were eliminated. She was able to walk, jump, and even skip rope.

SPINAL CORD INJURY

Another enigma that has eluded modern medicine, is the fact that a person having completely severed his/her spinal cord, still feels terrible pain below the level of the spinal cord injury (SCI). C. Nepomuceno, M.D., documented that 65 percent of people with spinal cord injury experienced pain within six months post injury, and 90 percent within four years.[21] There have been various names for this phenomenon including Central Dysesthesia Syndrome (dysesthesia means burning pain) or Central Pain Syndrome. I call it the "burning rectum syndrome" as the pain most often manifests in or near the rectum.

TRADITIONAL APPROACHES TO SCI PAIN MANAGEMENT

Whatever the name, many people with spinal cord injury have significant pain below the level of their SCI. The pain is similar to RSD pain and may radiate up or down the leg, but almost always resides in the rectal and pelvic area. Generally, traditional medical therapy provides only limited benefit. Eventually the person becomes addicted to narcotic medicines requiring larger doses to ease the pain. The medical personnel may become discouraged with the patient because of the continual requests for narcotics to control the pain. Soon the patient is labeled a drug addict.

More invasive approaches to control the pain include placement of a pump into the spinal canal which directly supplies narcotics into the spinal cord. Another approach is placing a spinal cord stimulator next to the spinal cord to "trick" the body so it does not feel the pain. The body, however, is smarter than any computer gizmo and the pain soon returns. Some people have resorted to having their spinal cord severed to relieve the pain. These treatments provide only temporary relief because they do not address the root cause of the problem. Chronic pain is never due to a narcotic deficiency, spinal cord stimulator implant deficiency, or a surgery deficiency. Chronic pain has a definite cause and until that cause is corrected, all other treatments are doomed to provide only temporary relief.

AUTONOMIC NERVOUS SYSTEM

The key to understanding the pain of spinal cord injury is the same as for Reflex Sympathetic Dystrophy: the autonomic nervous system. The autonomic nervous system is made up of two branches, the sympathetic nervous system which stimulates, and the parasympathetic nervous system which calms.

The sympathetic nerves reside in the spinal cord from T1 to L2.[22] This means the ganglia, the main control centers of the sympathetic nerves, travel from thoracic vertebrae number 1 to the lumbar vertebrae number two. If a person has a spinal cord lesion at the T6 level or above, when the sympathetic nervous system is stimulated, the body cannot shut it off automatically. For instance, if a person has a complete SCI at T5, and their foley catheter designed to drain their bladder clogs, the sympathetic nervous system would overactivate producing muscle spasticity, discrete body sweating (primarily above the lesion), and a significant rise in blood pressure. The brain senses the high blood pressure and sends parasympathetic stimulation through the spinal cord. This causes the heart rate to slow. The parasympathetic stimulation is not able to dilate the blood vessels in the abdomen or lower extremity because the nerve impulse stops at the T4 spinal cord injury. If the situation is not addressed, the result may be stroke or death. This condition is known as autonomic hyperreflexia.[23]

Although bladder distention is the most frequent stimulus in the production of autonomic hyperreflexia, doctors Head and Riddoch noted, "There is scarcely a stimulus, cutaneous, proprioceptive, or visceral, that may not be followed by an outburst of sweating appropriate to the lesion in each case."[24] In other words, sympathetic stimulation can occur from many different etiologies including ligament and tendon injury. It has been discussed how sympathetic hyperactivity can lead to burning pain, as in the case of reflex sympathetic dystrophy. Inflammation inside or around a joint can also lead to an increase in sympathetic tone.[25,26,27,28] If a joint or ligament is attempting to repair itself, the sympathetic nervous system may fire. If it continues, the condition becomes chronic. Chronic burning rectal or pelvic pain in an SCI patient is most often from chronic ligament or tendon laxity in the pelvis.

CAUSE OF SCI PAIN

A weakened ligament naturally tries to repair itself. Joint inflammation from a chronically weak ligament may be a cause for a hyperactive sympathetic system. This may lead to burning pain around the joint inflammation. As with RSD, the burning pain typically starts around the site of the initial injury.

People with complete SCIs cannot move their muscles below the level of the SCI. Because the muscles are paralyzed, the work of the ligaments to stabilize the joint is tremendously increased. The sacroiliac ligaments incur the greatest stress because sitting and sleeping positions necessitate pelvic stabilization. The ligamentous support of the pelvis and sacroiliac joint is at risk for injury during transfer, as in moving from a wheelchair to a bed.

Eventually, the sacroiliac, iliolumbar, sacrotuberous, and sacrospinous ligaments become lax. A well-known cause of coccygodynia (rectal pain) is injury to the sacrococcygeal joint. Coccygodynia is characterized by burning rectal pain. The onset of the pain is sudden, exquisite, and tender to palpation. Pain on movement of the coccyx is characteristic, meaning patients have pain when sitting or changing position.[29]

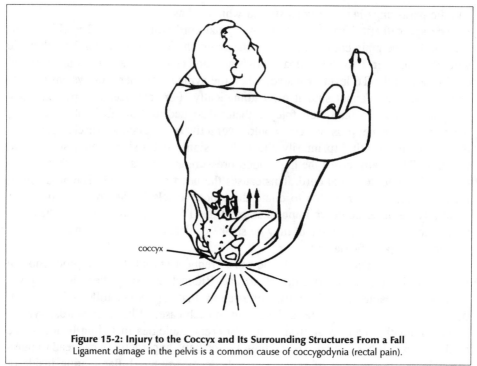

Figure 15-2: Injury to the Coccyx and Its Surrounding Structures From a Fall
Ligament damage in the pelvis is a common cause of coccygodynia (rectal pain).

COCCYGODYNIA (RECTAL PAIN)

Acute coccygodynia is most often caused by trauma to the coccyx and its surrounding structures, usually due to falling while in the half-seated position. **(Figure 15-2)** The coccyx itself is a bony structure attached to the end of the sacrum and is composed of three to five segments. The first and second segments may be separated by an intervertebral disc, but more commonly the segments are fused. The mobility, however, between the first and second segments predisposes this segment of the coccyx to fracture and dislocate.[30]

On the other hand, chronic coccygodynia is most commonly due to faulty posture while sitting or trauma to the coccyx during childbirth. Sitting in the slouched position puts stress on the coccyx rather than on the ischial tuberosities. **(Figure 15-3)** Other possible causes for coccygeal pain are chronic infection and dysfunction of the musculature of the pelvic floor.

People without SCI, who experience rectal pain, typically elicit a positive "jump sign" when the sacrococcygeal ligament is palpated. Prolotherapy to this ligament is curative in most cases. Some patients may also have laxity in the sacroiliac joint which requires treatment to resolve the chronic rectal pain.

The presentation of symptoms of coccygodynia in people without spinal cord injury and the dysesthetic syndrome that occurs in people with SCI are almost identical.

Traditional medical treatments for burning rectal pain include various medica-

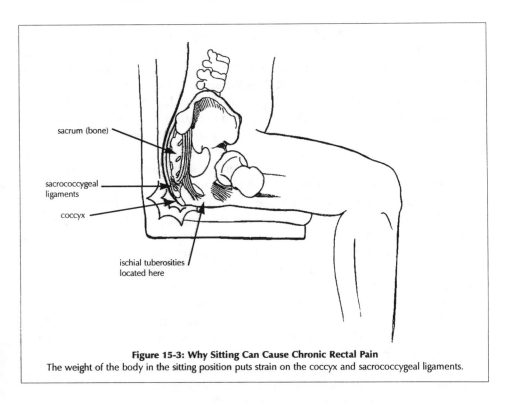

Figure 15-3: Why Sitting Can Cause Chronic Rectal Pain
The weight of the body in the sitting position puts strain on the coccyx and sacrococcygeal ligaments.

tions, physical therapy, seat cushions, and psychological support. These treatments typically provide only temporary benefit. Prolotherapy injections which strengthen the supporting structures of the sacrococcygeal joint eliminates chronic rectal pain because they address the root cause of the problem. Chronic rectal pain from coccygodynia occurs because of a weakness in the sacrococcygeal joint or a weakness between one of the coccygeal segments. Prolotherapy to strengthen the ligamentous support of the weakened area cures chronic rectal pain from coccygodynia.

CASE STUDY

Mike, a complete SCI patient at the fourth thoracic vertebrae level with a stabilizing rod placed in his spine from T2 to T7, suffered a T9 vertebral compression fracture. The surgeons wanted to put another rod down the rest of his vertebrae, but he heard about Prolotherapy and wanted a second opinion before being subjected to the knife. He was a wise man. All wise people with chronic pain obtain a consultation with a physician familiar with Prolotherapy.

He described his most distressing problem as constant burning rectal pain. Because he had no feeling below the level of his spinal cord lesion, it was not possible to elicit a positive "jump sign." Prolotherapy was performed on his thoracic spine and pelvic region.

When he returned for the second Prolotherapy session, he excitedly said, "Look, doc" and proceeded to bend forward on his wheelchair without the aid of a back brace. He previously required a back brace to support his thoracic spine while sitting. He lifted his hands perpendicular to the floor as he bent forward in his chair stating he was not able to do this prior to the first Prolotherapy treatment. It was also interesting that prior to the first Prolotherapy treatment, the physicians taking care of him told him he needed the surgery to stabilize his spine. I even spoke with his primary physician, a fellow Physiatrist, and explained it would be reasonable for him to try Prolotherapy to stabilize his spine, and that all conservative treatments should be exhausted prior to any surgical intervention. The Physiatrist had to approve the Prolotherapy for Mike in order to obtain insurance coverage. The Physiatrist would not consent but Mike decided to have the Prolotherapy and pay for it out of his own pocket. Mike's primary physician was so amazed when Mike returned for a follow-up visit after the first Prolotherapy session, that he recommended the insurance company pay for the Prolotherapy. Not only did they pay for the first Prolotherapy treatment, they agreed to pay for five more treatments.

I did not hear from Mike after his second session of Prolotherapy treatments so I phoned him. He exclaimed, "Doc, you know that rectal pain I was having all those years, well, I don't have that anymore!" This was amazing! After years of medicines, therapies, and cushions, two Prolotherapy treatments and Mike's dysesthetic syndrome was gone. How about his thoracic compression fracture? It has been 18 months since I first saw him and it has not deteriorated.

Most physicians desire what is best for their patients. Unfortunately, they do not know or understand all the treatment opinions. That is why each individual must take it upon themselves to explore all the treatment options. This is especially true prior to agreeing to the knife treatment.

VERTEBRAL COMPRESSION FRACTURES

Because people with complete SCI have no muscle movements below the level of the injury, severe osteoporosis is common. Osteoporosis is the main cause of vertebral compression fractures. Weakened bones cause a weakness in the fibro-osseous junction contributing to ligament and tendon laxity.[31] This laxity decreases the stability of the bones, especially around the vertebrae. Eventually because of the osteoporosis and the weakened ligaments, the vertebrae can no longer support the weight of the body and are compressed. This compressing of the vertebrae is known as a vertebral compression fracture. Prolotherapy helps stabilize the fracture site by causing the growth of ligament tissue at the fibro-osseous junction and strengthens the vertebral ligaments to eliminate the pain.

NEUROMAS

Burning pains in other parts of the body are believed to be due to nerve injuries or nerve tumors called "neuromas." Conventional treatments include blocking the nerve impulses or removing the "neuromas." Some of these "neuromas" even have names. In the foot, it is called Morton's neuroma. Dr. Hemwall believes there is no such thing as a "neuroma." When surgically examined, no tumor of the nerve is found. Treatments such as surgery or nerve blocks for these so-called "neuromas" often provide temporary benefit but do not cure the underlying condition because the burning pain does not originate in the nerves. If its origin was in the nerves then blocking the nerves, burning the nerves, or taking the nerves out would have definitive results.

The most common reason for burning pain anywhere in the body is ligament laxity. Chronic ligament laxity causes the sensory nerve endings within the ligaments to fire, stimulating the sympathetic system to become hyperactive. This leads to the chronic burning pain that people experience. Only Prolotherapy will supply definitive results in eliminating this type of chronic burning pain anywhere in the body.

POST-STROKE PAIN

Strokes, medically known as cerebrovascular lesions, are a major cause of long lasting disability. One of the worst consequences that occurs after a stroke is severe burning pain on the side of the body affected by the stroke. This type of condition is also known as central pain syndrome, neurogenic pain, or thalamic pain syndrome.

A person who has lost external sensation in a limb, due to a nerve injury or stroke, may experience severe burning pain in the area. Why this occurs is still unknown, but is most likely due to a hyperactive autonomic nervous system. This explains why a limb that is completely paralyzed can experience severe pain.

The pain experienced is usually constant, spontaneous and can in many cases be increased by various stimuli such as movements, cold, or warmth. It is usually severe and incapacitating, as it burns, pricks, lacerates, or aches. Typical treatments include pain medicines, muscle relaxants, physical therapy, and various anti-depressant medicines.[32,33] Often the treatments provide minimal relief. A much more effective treatment is Prolotherapy.

An example of this is B.S., a 72-year-old who had a stroke one and a half years prior to his first visit with Dr. Hemwall. The stroke left him paralyzed on his left side where he experienced severe burning pain. He tried all of the above treatments without success. Dr. Hemwall treated him with Prolotherapy to the entire left side of his body and spine. B.S. had dramatic results. B.S. has had some recurrence of his pain necessitating an occasional Prolotherapy "touch-up."

Prolotherapy injections cause the start of ligament and tendon tissue growth. It must be the stimulation of this growth that is registered in the spinal cord and/or brain that shuts down the pain provoking stimulus. Since post-stroke or post-nerve injury pain syndromes have no real treatment, Prolotherapy is a wonderful treatment option that could have curative results. It is for this reason that many people with post-stroke pain are choosing to Prolo their pain away.

PHANTOM PAIN

Another fascinating pain syndrome is the so-called "phantom pain." Early in the 1900s the famous French surgeon, Ambroise Pare, wrote, "Truly, it is a thing wondrous, strange, and prodigious, which will scarce be credited, unless by such as have seen with their own eyes and heard with their own ears, the patients who many months after cutting away the leg, grievously complained that they yet felt exceed-

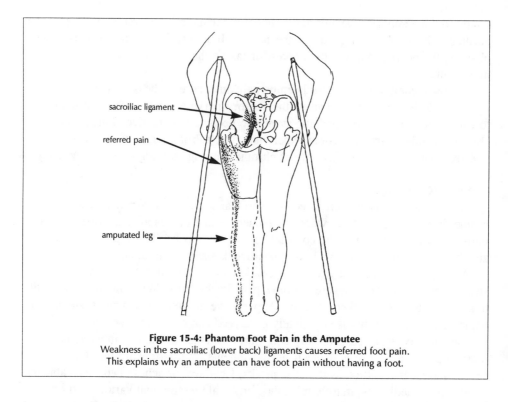

Figure 15-4: Phantom Foot Pain in the Amputee
Weakness in the sacroiliac (lower back) ligaments causes referred foot pain.
This explains why an amputee can have foot pain without having a foot.

ing great pain of that leg so cut off."[34]

Phantom sensation, phantom pain, or stump pain, occurs in people who have had an amputation, suffered a stroke, or paralysis of a section of the body. A weird sensation or pain is felt where the limb no longer exists or where there is no feeling. A typical scenario involves a gangrenous foot requiring amputation. Yes, some surgeries are necessary. After the surgery, some patients still experience the foot pain even though the foot is no longer there. **(Figure 15-4)**

Physicians will try anything to relieve the phantom pain. This includes the use of pain medicines, anti-convulsants, anti-depressants, nerve injections, prosthesis changes, physical therapy, and various "knife treatments" (surgeries). These treatments provide only temporary relief because they do not address the root cause of the problem.

The current theory on the development of phantom pain is that the absence of the limb or absence of sensation of the limb, causes an increase in nerve input from the brain to the limb. The additional nerve input causes the weird sensations and pain, but since the limb is absent, there is no system to deactivate the impulse.[35]

Dr. Hemwall, in the early 1970s treated a patient with terrible foot pain. Much to his surprise, upon examination, he had no foot! The person had an amputation of the leg years before. Nothing eased the pain he had. Dr. Hemwall knew that a common cause of foot pain was a referral pain from sacroiliac ligament laxity. He used his MRI (his thumb) and elicited a positive "jump sign" at the sacroiliac ligament.

Dr. Hemwall treated him with Prolotherapy. This patient with the terrible phantom pain became the first person healed of this condition through the use of Prolotherapy. Since that time, many others have had their phantom pains permanently eliminated with Prolotherapy.

Sacroiliac ligament laxity with referral pain to the foot, does not have any origins in the foot. The foot pain is actually from the ligament laxity in the pelvis. Most physicians do not know the referral pain patterns of ligaments and thus do not check for ligament laxity in the pelvis in phantom pain patients.

Phantom pain occurs in patients with amputations, spinal cord injury, or strokes. These medical conditions put additional strain on the sacroiliac ligaments. The sacroiliac joints play a greater role in stabilizing the pelvis and eventually become lax. The lax sacroiliac or other pelvic ligaments cause a referral pattern down the limb which is known as phantom pain. (*See Figure 15-4.*) Prolotherapy is very effective in treating this condition.

SUMMARY

Chronic burning pain from reflex sympathetic dystrophy, coccygodynia, neuromas, and spinal cord injury are often not due to a nerve injury. This is why typical treatments such as nerve blocks, medicines, and surgical procedures aimed at the nerves provide only temporary relief. Chronic burning pains, anywhere in the body, are usually caused by chronic ligament laxity. Prolotherapy causes a strengthening of the ligaments and has the potential to permanently eliminate dysesthetic syndromes which cause severe burning in the extremities. Because of this fact, many individuals are choosing to Prolo their RSD, SCI, and other neurological pains away.

CHAPTER 16

Prolo Your Unusual Pains Away

W hether someone says their back hurts, their chest hurts, or their tush hurts, most of us get tired of hearing them complain. More often than not, their back, chest, or tush really does hurt. People often have very unusual pain complaints. The more doctors people see for a pain complaint, the more likely their pain is real.

Unusual pain complaints are also a sign of ligament weakness. Even while at rest, a ligament can tense and cause pain, which explains how a person who is just sitting or lying down can have pain. Don't be too quick to call a spouse, brother, or friend "nutso" because of their pain. An evaluation by a physician experienced in Prolotherapy to look for ligament weakness and a positive "jump sign" should first be conducted. If ligament laxity can be found, most of their unusual pain complaints can be eliminated with Prolotherapy.

Pregnancy back pain, spastic torticollis, osteoporosis, cancer bone pain, and other unusual pains can be effectively treated with Prolotherapy.

BACK PAIN OF PREGNANCY

Steve, a pilot for a major airline carrier, arranged his schedule to fly into Chicago in order to receive Prolotherapy. Steve had what he termed "you name it, it hurts" syndrome. He had more surgeries on his TMJ than the Chicago Cubs have had losing seasons. He had benign congenital hypermobility, a condition found in only five percent of the population. With this condition, a person is born with unusually weak or lax ligaments. This makes them more prone to chronically loose joints and subsequent chronic pain. Because all of his joints were loose due to lax ligaments, every joint area of his body needed to be strengthened with Prolotherapy injections. Needless to say, Steve's treatments were quite extensive. His body responded wonderfully to the treatment, and after his third treatment his chiropractor noted that most of his vertebral segments were now stable.

What does this have to do with back pain of pregnancy, you ask? Steve's wife, Angie, accompanied him on his fourth visit. Angie had her own story to tell. She experienced terrible back pain while pregnant with their second child and vowed that she would never have another child. She explained that the back pain started with her pregnancy and continued to plague her after the baby was born.

I asked Angie on which hip she carried her baby. She told me it was the left hip.

I then asked her what side of her back hurt. Again, the answer was the left.

During pregnancy, women develop a positive "basketball-belly sign." This type of "basketball-belly sign" is permissible. During pregnancy, a woman's body secretes a hormone called relaxin, which causes ligaments to loosen allowing the baby to pass through the birth canal. Ligament laxity is normal during pregnancy. The baby's position in the pelvic region during pregnancy, the lax ligaments to allow delivery, and the mother carrying her baby on her hip after the baby is born all contribute to a resultant sacroiliac laxity and lower back pain.

In 1942, William Mengert, M.D., wrote, "It is now generally accepted that the overwhelming majority of backaches and sciaticas during pregnancy are due to pelvic girdle relaxation."[1] The average mobility of the joint is increased by 33 percent leading to lax ligaments in people experiencing back pain from the sacroiliac joint.[2]

Angie, seeing firsthand her husband's positive response to Prolotherapy, decided to try the treatment for her lower back pain. I warned her that a possible side effect of relief from her back pain would be a desire to have more children. After her first treatment, 50 percent of her back pain was alleviated.

When Angie came for her second treatment, she asked if the back pain would return with another pregnancy. I told her that Prolotherapy causes permanent strengthening of the ligaments and she could have all the children she wanted without fear of recurrent back pain. If some of her pain did return, however, a "touch-up" treatment would be all that was necessary. I also told her that if she did have another baby she should name him Ross. I did not hear from her for some time. Steve then called and announced they had another baby girl. Angie remained pain-free. Joyce Ann is the baby's name, although to me she will always be Ross, or at least Rose.

I also told Angie that her hips are not wide for carrying a baby on them, but are wide to get a baby out! A woman should never carry a baby on her hip. Many months are required after pregnancy for the sacroiliac joints to regain normal strength. It is imperative not to place any undue stress on the hips during this time. In Angie's case, carrying her first baby on her left hip was causing additional stress on the left sacroiliac joint. Her sacroiliac joints were already loose and painful during pregnancy. The addition of carrying a child on the hip after pregnancy did not give the sacroiliac joint a chance to heal. She then developed chronic sacroiliac laxity and its accompanying buddy, back pain. Prolotherapy in her case was curative and another wonderful life entered the world. **(Figure 16-1)**

Prolotherapy is an excellent treatment for back pain caused by pregnancy. Prolotherapy strengthens joints to relieve back pain but does not interfere with the birthing process. Prolotherapy has definitive results and can make pregnancy much more bearable. Prolotherapy is the treatment of choice for chronic low back pain that may occur during or linger after pregnancy if all other conservative treatments have proven unsuccessful.

SPASTIC TORTICOLLIS

Joan struggled with spastic torticollis for several years prior to coming to my office. Spastic torticollis is a condition in which the head will twitch or turn uncontrollably and

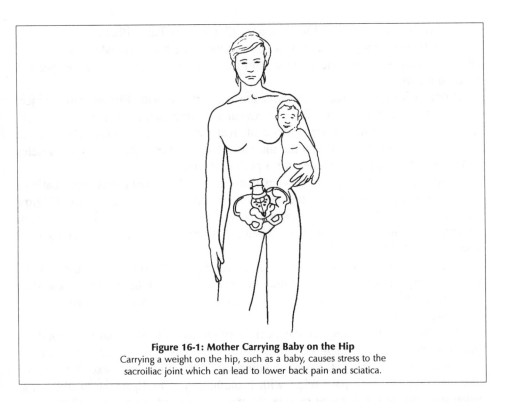

Figure 16-1: Mother Carrying Baby on the Hip
Carrying a weight on the hip, such as a baby, causes stress to the
sacroiliac joint which can lead to lower back pain and sciatica.

tilt to one side. Joan needed to turn her body to the side in order to see straight ahead. In addition to the social stigma, she experienced debilitating neck pain. Her attempts to relieve her pain with physical therapy, muscle relaxants, and Valium had proved unsuccessful. Spastic torticollis is not due to a Valium deficiency. Joan had heard about Prolotherapy and wanted to give it a try.

Like all chronic painful conditions, spastic torticollis has a cause, which is typically ligament laxity. Spastic torticollis causes involuntary muscle spasms in the neck.[3] The muscle spasms cause the neck to continually jerk the head to one side. Eventually, because the muscles continue to tighten, it becomes impossible to turn the head to the side.

Upon examining Joan, a positive "jump sign" was elicited when the cervical vertebral ligaments were palpated. Her twitching neck made the treatment difficult, but with persistence it was successfully completed. After the second treatment, Joan reported that she could sleep facing to the left.

Joan came all the way to Illinois from Tennessee to receive her treatment. When she heard I was going to be in South Carolina for a conference, she and a friend waited at my hotel for me to arrive. My hotel room was quickly converted into an examining room. I have given Prolotherapy treatments in churches, schools, homes, and hotels all around the country. I have given them on couches, beds, kitchen tables, the floor, dining room tables, and occasionally on examining room tables. My wife and I carry Prolotherapy supplies with us whenever we travel. Occasionally

I also give Prolotherapy treatments at my office in Oak Park, Illinois.

After five treatments, Joan was a new woman. She was fortunate to have heard about Prolotherapy. She had become pain-free, with the ability to turn her head in both directions.

People with spastic torticollis who are not familiar with Prolotherapy subject themselves to a series of painful and noncurative treatments. Surgery to cut tight muscles used to be the standard mode of treatment. The latest treatment involves injecting the botulism toxin into the muscles. The toxin paralyzes the tight muscles and allows the head to straighten for a period of time.

Similar to the case of reflex sympathetic dystrophy, spastic torticollis patients will often describe an injury to the neck prior to the onset of the condition. **(Figure 16-2)** It is advisable that a person with spastic torticollis receive an evaluation from a physician familiar with Prolotherapy before undergoing surgery or receiving toxin injections.

Once a ligament is loose, as occurs in a neck injury, the overlying muscles must tighten to support the structure. If only one side of the neck ligaments loosen, then the muscles on that side of the neck will become spastic. This is how spastic torticollis may form.

If significant shortening of the neck muscles has already occurred, botulism injections may be helpful in conjunction with Prolotherapy. If shortening of the muscles has not occurred, the person with spastic torticollis has an excellent chance to have complete neck pain relief with Prolotherapy. The ligaments in the neck, when strengthened, will cause muscle spasms to cease and allow the neck to regain full range of motion. Prolotherapy will terminate the chronic neck pain from spastic torticollis because it addresses the root cause of the problem.

OSTEOPOROSIS AND COMPRESSION FRACTURES

The problems associated with osteoporosis keep many doctors in business. Children drinking soda pop, eating candy, and chomping on potato chips make good prospects for future osteoporosis patients; all these contribute to the onset of this disease. This is due to the inadequate amount of calcium, magnesium, and vitamin D in these so-called foods. (A more appropriate name for these items would be edible chemicals.) The phosphorus from soda pop actually leaches calcium out of the bone, making eventual osteoporosis very likely.

An estimated 1.2 million osteoporotic fractures occur annually and more than half occur in the vertebrae.[4] The incidence of osteoporosis is directly correlated to testosterone production in men and estrogen and progesterone production in women. Women are especially at risk after menopause because of the drastic cessation of hormone production, whereas men experience a more gradual decline in hormone production as they age.

I recommend that all women take natural hormone replacements at the start of menopause and see a Natural Medicine physician for a natural health maintenance program. (*See Appendix C, Natural Medicine Resources.*) Exercise, calcium, magnesium, a healthy diet, and natural hormones are excellent ways for women to keep

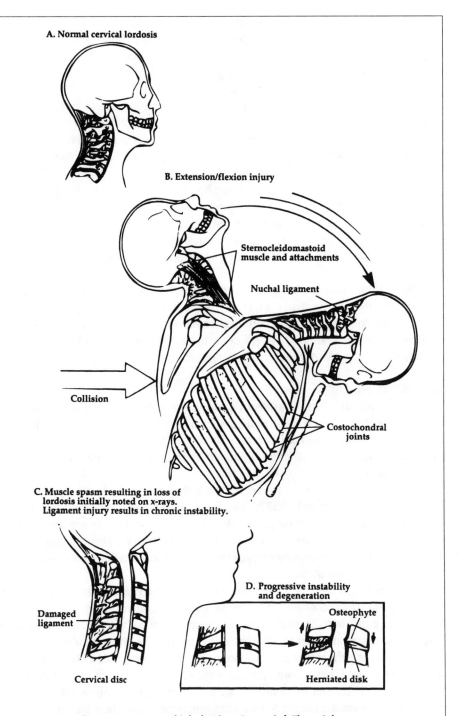

A. Normal cervical lordosis

B. Extension/flexion injury

Sternocleidomastoid muscle and attachments

Nuchal ligament

Collision

Costochondral joints

C. Muscle spasm resulting in loss of lordosis initially noted on x-rays. Ligament injury results in chronic instability.

Damaged ligament

Cervical disc

D. Progressive instability and degeneration

Osteophyte

Herniated disk

Figure 16-2: How a Whiplash Injury Causes Soft Tissue Injury
Nonhealed soft tissue injury can eventually lead to conditions such as arthritis and spastic torticollis.

Ligament and Tendon Relaxation Treated by Prolotherapy © 1991, Gustav A. Hemwall, M.D. Used with permission.

their bones strong and maintain a zest for life.

Osteoporosis may cause vertebral compression, a painful and disabling condition. A vertebral compression fracture will normally occur in the thoracic or lumbar region of the back. Untreated compression fractures from osteoporosis in the thoracic region may lead to a humpback deformity.[5]

The mainstay treatment for a vertebral compression fracture is wearing a brace to properly position the back while the fracture heals. The problem with this treatment is that the vertebral fractures from osteoporosis are not a back brace deficiency. Thus, this type of treatment, even if exercise and nonsteroidal anti-inflammatory agents are added for good measure, does not cure the underlying cause of the problem.

Prolotherapy, in strengthening the fibro-osseous junction, the ligament-bony interface, permanently stabilizes the compressed vertebral segment. The strengthening of the ligament and periosteal interface realign the area resulting in improved posture. Prolotherapy, however, is not a complete treatment for osteoporosis compression fractures. The underlying cause must be corrected or the osteoporosis will recur.

Whether the cause is nutritional, hormonal, or a chronic disease, the underlying etiology of the osteoporosis must be addressed to ensure long-term healing. Prolotherapy to strengthen the vertebral supporting ligaments, in conjunction with Natural Medicine treatments, is effective in healing the pain and disability caused by osteoporosis-induced vertebral compression fractures.

CANCER BONE PAIN

People with all different kinds of chronic diseases and many different kinds of pain syndromes visit Caring Medical and Rehabilitation Services, S.C., the Natural Medicine clinic my wife and I operate. Some patients at the clinic are trying Natural Medicine techniques in order to stimulate their immune systems and enable their bodies to fight cancer.

Cancer, by definition, is a group of cells that say to the body, "I'm the boss." The cancer cells grow and steal blood, blood vessels, and nutrients from the body, invading any area where they can grow. Many pain syndromes are associated with cancer, but the most severe pain occurs when the cancer invades the bone. Traditional treatments for cancer pain include narcotic medications or some type of radioactivity directed at the cancer site.[6,7]

Cancer does not usually cause bone pain until the outside of the bone, the periosteum, is cracked. The inside of the bone does not contain nerve endings and thus cannot feel pain, but the outside of the bone is loaded with nerve endings.[8] This helps explain why injuries at the fibro-osseous junction are so painful.

Cancer bone pain is brutal, often requiring high doses of narcotic medications to relieve the pain. Unfortunately, these high doses of medications leave a person dependent on drugs and in an altered state. Treatments that allow for a decrease in the amount of narcotic medications would greatly improve the cancer patient's quality of life.

In the early 1960s, Marsha, a four-year post-mastectomy patient, visited Dr.

Hemwall because of dull back pain. Dr. Hemwall treated her mid-back region with Prolotherapy. He instructed her to have the area X-rayed and follow up with her primary physician. Several years later, Dr. Hemwall learned that at the time he treated her, Marsha had a recurrence of breast cancer, according to the X-ray. Interestingly, the Prolotherapy treatment had eliminated Marsha's bone pain from the cancer and greatly improved her quality of life. This was the first of five cases where Dr. Hemwall used Prolotherapy to eliminate cancer bone pain.

Prolotherapy is helpful in eliminating or diminishing cancer bone pain because strengthening the area, the fibro-osseous junction, causes the nerve endings in the periosteum to stop firing. Prolotherapy does not affect the underlying cancerous condition. The etiological basis for the cancer must be corrected whether a person decides to use traditional medical treatments or Natural Medicine treatments. Prolotherapy is an effective tool to assist with pain from cancer invading the bone.

BUTTOCK PAIN

Some people experience pain in the posterior, while others are a pain in the posterior. When you sit down, your tush normally rests on the ischial tuberosity. Since many of us have sedentary jobs and buttocks that are a few sizes too big, the soft tissue surrounding the ischial tuberosity bones is compressed. The structures that attach to the ischial tuberosity are the sacrotuberous ligaments and the hamstring muscles. **(Figure 16-3)**

The most common cause of pain at the cheek line in the buttock area is weakness in the structures that attach to the ischial tuberosity. The condition that is manifested by buttock pain and tenderness over the ischial tuberosity is known in traditional medical lingo as ischial bursitis. A bursa is a fluid-filled sac that allows tendons and muscles to glide over the bones. Bursitis means inflammation of the bursa. True bursitis pain is so painful that any pressure to the bursa would elicit a positive "hit the ceiling" sign. True bursitis is extremely rare. If a physician diagnoses bursitis and recommends a cortisone shot to relieve the inflammation, I recommend a fast exit out the door. Remember, chronic pain is not due to a cortisone deficiency and is rarely due to bursitis.

Prolotherapy injections for buttock pain are given all along the ischial tuberosity, where the hamstring muscles and sacrotuberous ligaments attach. Prolotherapy will strengthen this area. This is another area that is rarely examined by a traditional physician. I do not think any one of my patients has told me that any other doctor has examined their ischial tuberosities. After four sessions of Prolotherapy, the buttock pain is usually eliminated.

RECTAL, VAGINAL, TESTICULAR, AND TAILBONE PAIN

It is amusing for me to hear the diagnoses people have been given for their conditions. Just recently, a patient told me she had vulvodynia. She was very happy that someone had finally given her a diagnosis for her pain. She was crushed when I told her this meant vaginal pain. Vulva means vaginal and dynia means pain. All the doctor did was tell her something she already knew. She had vaginal pain. Diagnoses

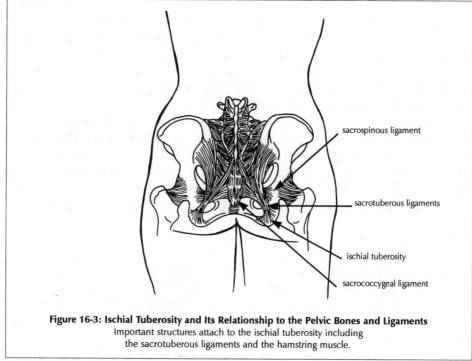

Figure 16-3: Ischial Tuberosity and Its Relationship to the Pelvic Bones and Ligaments
Important structures attach to the ischial tuberosity including
the sacrotuberous ligaments and the hamstring muscle.

Ligament and Tendon Relaxation Treated by Prolotherapy © 1991, Gustav A. Hemwall, M.D. Used with permission.

like lumbago or lumbalgia (back pain), cervicalgia (neck pain), fibromyalgia (body pain), or proctalgia (rectal pain) are not diagnoses. They are terms for the symptoms.

Roughly 15 percent of the population at one time or another will experience rectal pain which is commonly diagnosed as proctalgia or proctalgia fugax.[9] It is characterized by episodic sharp pain in the rectal region, lasting for several seconds to several minutes. Traditional treatments include pain medications, steroid injections, counseling, or biofeedback.[10] Since no standard medical treatment is very effective, both the physician and the patient are easily frustrated. Often the patient is labeled as having irritable bowel syndrome, again a fancy diagnosis which just labels the symptoms.

Rectal, vaginal, testicular, or tailbone pain, like pain anywhere else in the body, has a cause. Generally, these pains can be reproduced when the ligaments around the pelvis are palpated. The most commonly affected areas are the ligaments around the sacrococcygeal junction which includes the sacrococcygeal ligament, sacrotuberous, and sacrospinous ligaments. **(Figure 16-3)** Since these ligaments are near the rectum, it makes sense that rectal or groin pains originate from these structures. When Prolotherapy has strengthened these ligaments, chronic rectal pain dissipates.

Another common cause of chronic groin, testicular, or vaginal pain is iliolumbar ligament weakness because this ligament refers pain from the lower back to these areas. Prolotherapy of the iliolumbar ligament can be curative for chronic groin, testicular, or vaginal pain. **(Figure 16-4)**

D.B., a 45-year-old gentleman, went to see Bernadette Kohn, M.D., because of severe burning pain near the rectum. His job entailed extensive traveling and his pain made sitting nearly impossible. After sitting for five minutes, the pain, which he described as a "burning poker up you know where" would hit. He endured two back surgeries with only minor relief of his pain. He even went to a well-known clinic where he was told the "scar tissue" from his previous surgeries was causing his pain. He was advised to live with the pain.

Live with the pain?! Hogwash! Who wants to live with pain?! Fortunately for D.B., he consulted a physician trained in Prolotherapy. His first Prolotherapy treatment enabled D.B. to travel for more than two hours without pain in his tailbone area. Dr. Kohn reported that D.B. was extremely grateful for the Prolotherapy treatment he received.

Chronic rectal or tailbone pain can be horribly disabling as this case illustrates. After extensive testing, patients are often given dubious diagnoses such as proctalgia fugax, anorectal neuralgia, levator ani syndrome, coccygodynia, or spastic pelvic floor syndrome.[11,12,13,14] Typical conservative traditional treatments include pain medicines, sitz baths (sitting in a hot tub), local anesthetic creams, massage, muscle relaxants, electrical stimulation gizmos, or the end-all pain treatment, an anti-depressant medication. Such treatments generally have unsatisfactory results because they do not correct the underlying cause of the chronic rectal pain.

As in other parts of the body, the most important evaluation in analyzing chronic rectal pain is palpation of the area. A positive "jump sign" can typically be elicited by palpation of the sacrococcygeal ligaments. If no "jump sign" is elicited, then the other pelvic ligaments are palpated, such as the sacrotuberous, sacrospinous, iliolumbar, and sacroiliac ligaments. When a positive "jump sign" is elicited over the painful ligament, both the patient and the doctor know that the cause of the pain is a weakened ligament.

A weakened sacrococcygeal ligament is stretched even further when a person has a bowel movement or sits. (*Refer to Figure 15-3.*) People with chronic rectal or tailbone pain often have an increase in pain upon performing these tasks. The best treatment for a weakened ligament is Prolotherapy. Prolotherapy treatments to the weakened pelvic ligaments help these areas heal and return to normal strength. Once the sacrococcygeal, iliolumbar, and other weakened pelvic ligaments are strong again, the chronic rectal pain abates. This is why many people with chronic rectal, tailbone, groin, testicular, and vaginal pains are choosing to Prolo their pain away.

SLIPPING RIB SYNDROME

Dawn, a 35-year-old, was rushed to the hospital for the fourth time in less than a year complaining of severe chest pain, fearing a heart attack. After EKGs, blood tests, X-rays, and a stay in the intensive care unit, the cause of her pain was still unknown. Everyone began to wonder if she was a little crazy.

As I examined her, Dawn initially explained that she was not currently having severe chest pain but did feel a dull ache in her chest. I told her she needed one more diagnostic test, the trusty MRI—**M**y **R**eproducibility **I**nstrument. In a second,

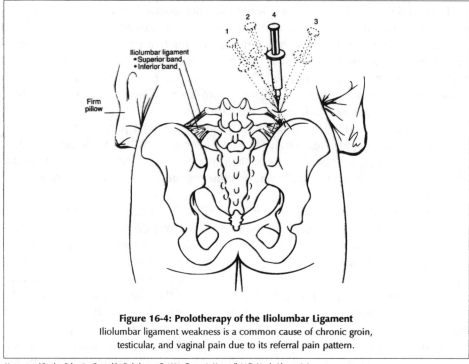

Figure 16-4: Prolotherapy of the Iliolumbar Ligament
Iliolumbar ligament weakness is a common cause of chronic groin,
testicular, and vaginal pain due to its referral pain pattern.

Ligament and Tendon Relaxation Treated by Prolotherapy © 1991, Gustav A. Hemwall, M.D. Used with permission.

the diagnosis was made. I pressed on her left fourth thoracic rib attachment onto the sternum and Dawn's severe crushing chest pain immediately returned. I asked her if she had ever been examined in this fashion. She said she had not. Dawn's pain was caused by Slipping Rib Syndrome.

An extremely important point illustrated by Dawn's case is that even if an X-ray, blood sample, or EKG does not reveal a cause, they do not eliminate the presence of a physical condition as the source of chest pain. It is much more likely that the chronic chest pain is due to weakened soft tissue, such as a ligament or tendon. If heart and lung tests prove normal, yet the patient claims to be still experiencing pain, the patient is often diagnosed as being crazy. It is imperative for anyone given a psychiatric diagnosis as the basis for the chronic pain to have an evaluation by a physician competent in the treatment of Prolotherapy.

Depression, anxiety, and being a little crazy are not the etiological bases for most chronic pain. They can be associated factors involved in the problem, but they are normally not the cause. If depressed people complain of shoulder pain, most likely they have shoulder pain. Chronic pain should be assumed to be originating from a weakened soft tissue, such as a ligament or tendon. This condition should be treated with Prolotherapy before the diagnosis of "cuckoo" is made. A weak tendon, like the rotator cuff, or ligament, such as the coracoacromial ligament, may be the cause. If traditional treatments leave the patient with the impression that the pain is all psychological, then an evaluation by a Prolotherapist will save them from a

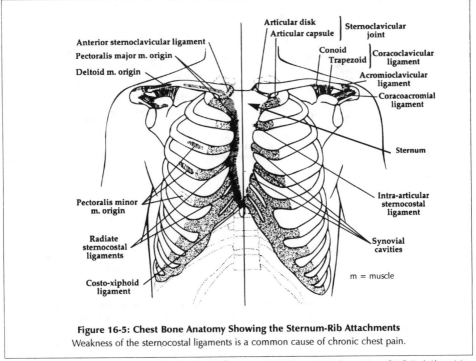

Figure 16-5: Chest Bone Anatomy Showing the Sternum-Rib Attachments
Weakness of the sternocostal ligaments is a common cause of chronic chest pain.

psychological stigma and a life of chronic pain. Dawn's pain was indeed real and it was eliminated by Prolotherapy.

Slipping Rib Syndrome, also known as Tietze's Syndrome, was first described in 1921 by Alexander Tietze, M.D., as chest pain over the sternoclavicular and costochondral junctions.[15] Other names include xiphoidalgia, costochondritis, or anterior chest-wall syndrome. But the most descriptive and accurate name for the actual etiological basis of the condition is Slipping Rib Syndrome.[16] It is interesting to note that just one year after Dr. Tietze's description, Slipping Rib Syndrome was described in medical literature.[17]

In Dawn's case, a rib was slipping out of place because the ligaments that hold the ribs to the sternum, the sternocostal ligaments, were weak. **(Figure 16-5)** Without muscles to hold the ribs in place, loose ligaments allow slipping of the rib which causes further stretching of the ligament, manifesting itself by producing severe pain. The loose ribs can also pinch intercostal nerves, sending excruciating pains around the chest into the back. Sternocostal and costochondral ligaments refer pain from the front of the chest to the mid back. Likewise, costovertebral ligament sprains refer pain from the back of the rib segment to the sternum where the rib attaches. **(Figures 16-6)**

Traditional medicine believes the condition is caused by inflammation in the costochondral junction causing costochondritis. The treatment of choice in traditional medical circles is, you guessed it, an NSAID, a nonsteroidal anti-inflammatory drug.

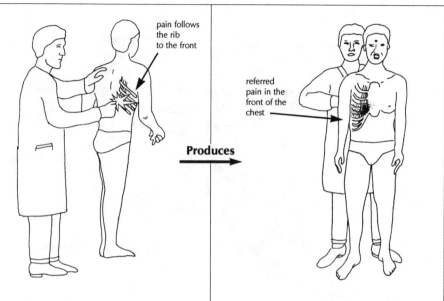

Figure 16-6A: Physician Reproduces Pain at the Rib-Vertebrae Junction
Weakness at the rib-vertebrae (costovertebral) junction ligaments are a common source of mid-back pain.

Figure 16-6B: Referral Pain Pattern of the Rib-Sternal Junction
Rib-vertebrae (costovertebral) ligament weakness can cause pain to occur in the chest.

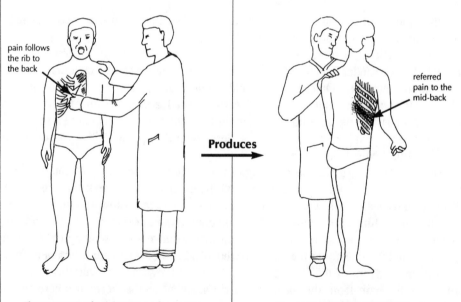

Figure 16-6C: Physician Reproduces Pain at the Rib-Sternal Junction
Weakness at the rib-sternal (costochondral or sternocostal) junction ligaments is a common source of chest pain.

Figure 16-6D: Referral Pain Pattern of the Rib-Vertebrae Junction
Rib-sternal (costochondral or sternocostal) ligament weakness can cause pain to occur in the side or mid-back region.

Chronic pain, no matter what the cause, is not due to a NSAID deficiency. Slipping Rib Syndrome is caused by weakness of the sternocostal, costochondral, or costovertebral ligaments. Prolotherapy will strengthen these ligament junctions in all the areas where the ribs are hypermobile.

Slipping Rib Syndrome may be caused by hypermobility of the anterior end of the costal cartilage, located at the rib-cartilage interface called the costochondral junction. Most often, the tenth rib is the source because, unlike ribs one through seven which attach to the sternum, the eighth, ninth, and tenth ribs are attached anteriorly to each other by loose, fibrous tissue.[18] This provides increased mobility, but a greater susceptibility to trauma. Slipping rib cartilage may cause no pain or only intermittent pain.[19]

Slipping Rib Syndrome is also more likely to occur in the lower ribs because of the poor blood supply to the cartilaginous tissue and ligaments. Injury to the cartilage tissue in the lower ribs or the sternocostal ligaments in the upper ribs seldom completely heal naturally. The sternocostal, rib-sternum, and costochondral joints undergo stress when the rib cage expands or contracts abnormally or when excessive pressure is applied on the ribs themselves.

In order for the rib cage to expand and contract with each breath, the costochondral and the sternocostal junctions are naturally loose. Humans breathe 12 times per minute, 720 times per hour, 19,280 times per day, which stresses these ligamentous-rib junctions. Additional stressors include any condition that makes breathing more difficult. A simple coughing attack due a cold may cause the development of Slipping Rib Syndrome. Conditions such as bronchitis, emphysema, allergies, and asthma cause additional stress to the sternocostal and costochondral junctions. Even sinusitis, with the associated nose blowing can be the initial event that leads to chronic chest pain from Slipping Rib Syndrome.

Other causes of Slipping Rib Syndrome include the feared "fall asleep in the back seat of a crowded car syndrome." A person falls asleep in a crowded car with the door handle jutting into a rib. The rib slips out of place and the problem begins. Another cause of Slipping Rib Syndrome is the result of surgery to the lungs, chest, heart, or breast with resection of the lymph nodes which puts a tremendous stress on the rib attachments because the surgeon must separate the ribs to remove the injured tissue. Unresolved chest or upper back pain following a thoracotomy, chest operation, or CPR is most likely due to ligament laxity in the rib-sternum or the rib-vertebral junction.

The ribs are attached in the front, as well as in the back of the body. A loose rib in the front is likely also loose in the back. The rib-vertebral junction is known as the costovertebral junction, and is secured by the costotransverse ligaments. Unexplained upper back pain, between the shoulder blades and costovertebral, rib-vertebrae pain, is likely due to joint laxity and/or weakness in the costotransverse ligaments. **(Figure 16-7)**

Chronic chest pain, especially in young people, is often due to weakness in the sternocostal and costochondral junctions, and chronic mid-upper back pain is due to weakness at the costovertebral junction. Both conditions may lead to Slipping Rib

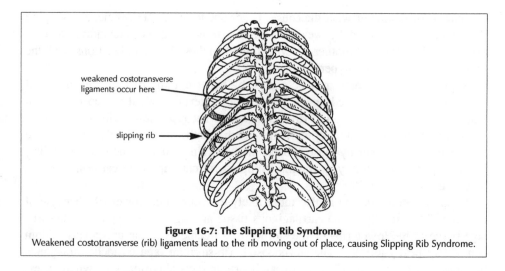

weakened costotransverse
ligaments occur here

slipping rib

Figure 16-7: The Slipping Rib Syndrome
Weakened costotransverse (rib) ligaments lead to the rib moving out of place, causing Slipping Rib Syndrome.

Syndrome where the rib intermittently slips out of place, causing a stretching of the ligamentous support of the rib in the front and back. The result is periodic episodes of severe pain and underlying chronic chest and/or upper back pain. Prolotherapy, by strengthening these areas, provides definitive results in the relief of the chronic chest pain or chronic upper back pain from Slipping Rib Syndrome.

ILIOCOSTALIS SYNDROME

Undiagnosed chronic side pain affects many people, occurring most often in people suffering from osteoporosis. Iliocostalis Syndrome, also known as iliocostal friction syndrome, is a condition caused by friction of the lower ribs against the iliac crest, leading to irritation of soft tissues.[20]

The distance between the lower ribs and iliac crest is normally sufficient to prevent contact, even when bending to the side. When the lower ribs of iliocostalis syndrome patients come into contact with the iliac crest, especially when side bending, friction and damage is caused to the tendons and muscles that insert at the iliac crest and the lower rib cage. **(Figure 16-8)**

The condition commonly occurs from a vertebral deformity such as scoliosis, disc degeneration, or the most common cause: vertebral compression fractures. This bone to bone contact manifests itself as back or side pain. Palpation along the iliac crest is usually painful but rarely elicits the classic positive "jump sign." A more definitive method of diagnosing the problem is feeling the contact of the ribs and the iliac crest upon bending to the side.

Prolotherapy will strengthen the muscles and tendons that insert onto the iliac crest and lower rib margins, as well as the fibro-osseous junction.[21] If the muscles and tendons are pinched when the bones collide, during side bending, they will have strength to tolerate the event after Prolotherapy; though it is recommended not to bend sideways to prevent the rib and pelvic bones from colliding. Prolotherapy is very effective in eliminating the chronic side pains caused by Iliocostalis Syndrome.

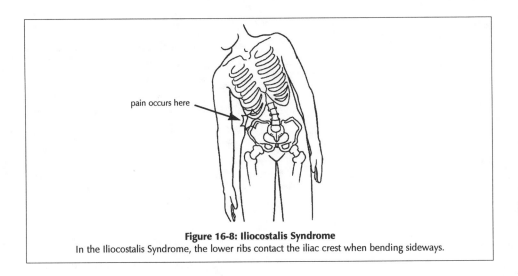

Figure 16-8: Iliocostalis Syndrome
In the Iliocostalis Syndrome, the lower ribs contact the iliac crest when bending sideways.

SUMMARY

Many chronic pain sufferers have not found relief with traditional medicine. When blood tests and X-rays do not reveal a cause, they are told their pain is psychological. Chronic pain is most often caused by ligament or tendon laxity. Prolotherapy is effective at eliminating chronic pain because it helps ligaments and tendons grow. Prior to agreeing with a psychological diagnosis for pain, or agreeing to surgery, I would advise that an evaluation be performed by a physician familiar with Prolotherapy.

The etiological basis for many unusual pain syndromes, such as spastic torticollis, cancer bone pain, ischial tendonitis, Slipping Rib Syndrome, vulvodynia, proctalgia fugax, coccygodynia, and Iliocostalis Syndrome is often due to a weakness at the fibro-osseous junction of soft tissue, such as a ligament or tendon. Chronic low back pain in pregnancy may be due to lax ligaments, specifically the sacroiliac ligaments. Prolotherapy injections stimulate the growth of ligament and tendon tissue at the fibro-osseous junction, strengthen the area and resolve the chronic pain syndrome. It is for this reason that many people are choosing to Prolo their unusual pain syndromes away.

CHAPTER 17

Prolo Your Sports Injuries Away

W hat do professional swimmers from France, basketball players from New Jersey, hockey players from Chicago, tennis players from Florida, and the thousands of so-called "weekend warriors" all have in common? At some point, while playing their sport of choice, they will each experience a sports injury.

Sports plays a very important role in American society. In addition to the income generated, sports is an outlet for amusement and exercise. Sports also provides an environment for both young and old to develop friendships and hopefully character.

Therefore, it is quite a dramatic event when an athlete is sidelined due to injury. Not being able to play sends many into a panic. Fearing they will never again experience the thrill of victory, athletes are willing to do almost anything to get back in the game. The thrill of victory is never forgotten once it has been tasted.

REASONS FOR SPORTS INJURIES

Most sports injuries are soft tissue injuries involving ligaments, tendons, and muscles.[1] Sports injuries occur when the repetitive strain of the athletic event is too much for a particular ligament, tendon, or muscle to withstand, resulting in a strain, an injured weakened tendon, or a sprain, an injured weakened ligament.

The customary treatment for such injuries, as discussed in Chapters Five and Six, is RICE which refers to treating soft injury tissue with Rest, Ice, Compression, and Elevation. This treatment regime decreases inflammation when the injured area needs it most, resulting, unfortunately for the athlete, in decreased healing of the injury. Consequently, many sports injuries do not heal completely and are easily re-injured.

A better approach is a treatment known as MEAT—Movement, Exercise, Analgesics, and Treatment. Specific treatments that aid in the healing process include ultrasound, heat, and massage because they increase blood flow. If an injury has not healed after six weeks, more aggressive treatments, including Prolotherapy, should be considered. Prolotherapy can be done immediately after an injury because it has been found to speed recovery.

Stretching, body balancing or body work, chiropractic or osteopathic manipulation, and other physical modalities do help correct problems with posture, tight muscles, and other factors that contribute to sports injuries. The fact remains that sports injuries occur when an area in the body is weak. Sports injuries, whether an ankle

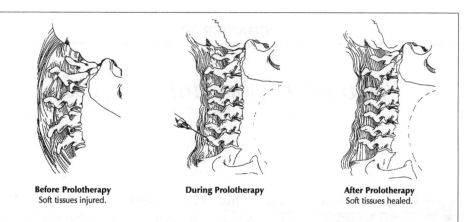

Before Prolotherapy
Soft tissues injured.

During Prolotherapy

After Prolotherapy
Soft tissues healed.

Figure 17-1: Prolotherapy Curing Neck Pain From Any Cause Including Sports Injury
Prolotherapy stimulates the growth of soft tissue, such as ligaments and tendons, relieving chronic neck pain.

sprain or rotator cuff tendonitis, occur because a muscle, ligament, or tendon is not strong enough to perform the task the athlete requires of it. For this reason, the best curative treatment for a sports injury is to strengthen the weakened tissue.

Many sports injuries are muscle strains. Such injuries cause muscle pain when the injured muscle is contracted. Muscles enjoy a constant blood supply which brings them necessary healing ingredients. As a result, muscles are usually quick to heal—regardless of the treatment.

As discussed in Chapter Six, ligaments and tendons have poor blood supply and are thus more prone to incomplete healing after an injury. The goal in sports injury therapy should not be pain relief but normal tissue strength, in other words complete healing of the injured body part. Unfortunately, most athletes are attended to by clinicians who provide pain relief in the form of ibuprofen, aspirin, cortisone shots, and surgery. These therapies can provide pain relief, but they do so at the expense of long-term weakened tissue. I believe most athletes want strong tissue, not weak tissue.

TREATMENT FOR SPORTS INJURIES

Prolotherapy is the best treatment to help cause permanently strong tissue to form where a weakened sports injury exists. Prolotherapy stimulates the healing process and therefore decreases the length of time it takes for soft tissue sports injuries to heal. Prolotherapy, because it triggers the growth of normal collagen tissue, causes stronger ligaments and tendons to form. **(Figure 17-1)** Consequently, the athlete returns to his game stronger. After Prolotherapy treatments not only is the athlete able to return to the sport, but often the particular area that was injured will be stronger than before the injury and performance will be enhanced.

FREQUENCY OF PROLOTHERAPY FOR SPORTS INJURIES

Because injured athletes often desire to return to their game as soon as possible, Prolotherapy injections may be given weekly instead of every six weeks. This is because athletes do not have the time to wait to grow tissue. They desire tissue growth and they want it now! Sometimes stronger solutions are used to help increase the speed of the healing process. This is not the ideal situation, however. A preferred treatment regime is for athletes to receive Prolotherapy treatments during their off season so that by the start of the season the injury is healed.

I have personally experienced the success of this treatment. I had habitual ankle sprains during my youth that prevented me from participating in several sports. Prolotherapy treatment on my ankles has enabled me to now participate in whatever sport I desire (with my wife's permission, of course). I also enjoy long-distance running and have completed one marathon and two half marathons in my lifetime, so I was quite frustrated when I recently found myself barely able to walk because of debilitating knee pain. My friend, Rodney Van Pelt, M.D., performed Prolotherapy on the cruciate ligaments in my knee. Only one treatment was necessary to put me back into my running shoes. I am currently training for a second marathon.

ROLE OF SURGERY IN SPORTS INJURIES

Gustav A. Hemwall, M.D., the world's most experienced Prolotherapist, and I have had professional as well as amateur athletes come through our office doors and, most importantly, leave and return to playing their sport. It saddens me when I read in the newspaper about a professional athlete undergoing surgery for a sports injury. The knife treatment often is equivalent to a death sentence for the professional athlete. Surgery often ends or severely limits their career.

Surgery weakens tissue. What do you think the doctor actually does when he or she says "I'm going to scope the knee"? "Scoping" involves removing a little tissue here, cutting a little tissue there. Frayed tissue is either shaved or cut out. Surgery for sports injuries, even arthroscopic surgery, means the surgeon is going to remove tissue. Realize that removing cartilage, ligament, or any other soft tissues of the body makes that body part weaker.

Rather than weakening their bodies with surgery, athletes should strengthen their bodies with Prolotherapy. Prolotherapy helps frayed, weakened tissue repair itself and makes that particular body part strong again. Surgery often spells death for an athlete. Prolotherapy spells new life!

SUMMARY

In summary, sports injuries are caused because muscle, tendon, or ligament tissue is too weak to perform a particular task. Treatment regimes for soft tissue injury, such as taking ibuprofen and applying ice to the area to reduce inflammation, or undergoing surgery to remove tissue, often provide pain relief but cause incomplete healing, making the athlete prone to re-injury.

A better approach to treatment of sports injuries, more than just pain control, is complete healing of the injured tissue. Prolotherapy, because it stimulates the growth of ligament and tendon tissue, helps sports injuries heal faster. While surgery causes tissue to become weaker, Prolotherapy helps form stronger tissue.

Because athletes desire to continue playing their sports without a reduction in ability or fear of reinjury, many are choosing to Prolo their sports injuries away.

CHAPTER 18

Prolo Your Animal's Pain Away

thought most pet owners were fanatical until Squeaky came on the scene. Squeaky is the cat my wife and I rescued from our farm home in southern Illinois. One weekend she was limping, so we decided to take her home to Oak Park, Illinois, to "rehabilitate" her. Once she was inside our warm home, she dramatically "healed." Whenever we talk about returning her to southern Illinois, her ailment strangely returns. It looks like she has become a permanent part of our family.

DUKE'S STORY

I understood his emotion when one of my Prolotherapy patients said to me sadly, "Duke cannot climb the stairs anymore."

He then asked, "Since Prolotherapy was so effective for me, will it work for my dog, Duke?"

Climbing the stairs was painful for Duke, just as it is for humans with joint pain.

I asked a veterinarian friend, Shaun Fauley, D.V.M., to assist me. Duke, a big, old dog was favoring his left leg which led us to believe his hip was the source of his pain. Dr. Fauley anesthetized Duke and we performed Prolotherapy on his left hip and pelvis. One hour later, Duke was up and running. The next day his limp had noticeably decreased. How could Duke have experienced such rapid pain relief?

The answer is the same for Duke as it is for humans. Two-thirds of patients (and animals) feel better immediately after the Prolotherapy treatment. The immediate inflammation caused by the Prolotherapy temporarily stabilizes the painful, loose joints. The new ligament and tendon tissue does not fully form for four to six weeks after the treatment. The time period between the reduction in inflammation and the fully formed tissue is a "window period" between the second and fourth week when the pain may return. **(Figure 18-1)** Complete healing occurs when the ligament and tendon tissue regains its normal strength. This normally requires four Prolotherapy sessions for humans. The time frame is less for animals.

In regard to Duke, after two months and one Prolotherapy session his overall function improved 50 percent. Many animals across the country are put to sleep—a gentle way of saying "killed"—because of their painful conditions. Even worse, there are many animals whose owners chase them so they can shove nonsteroidal anti-inflammatory drugs (NSAIDs), or other pain relievers down their throats to alleviate their pain. Animals are smarter than we are. They run from NSAIDs. We

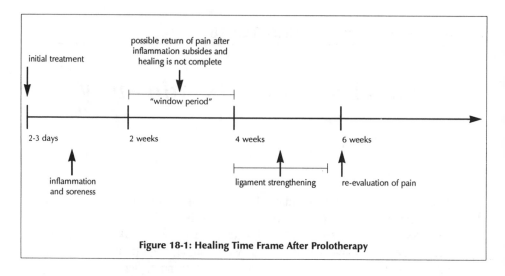

Figure 18-1: Healing Time Frame After Prolotherapy

humans run to NSAIDs.

Dr. Fauley and I treated Duke again with Prolotherapy injections in his left hip and pelvis. The last time I saw Duke, he was happily chasing birds.

PROLOTHERAPY IN VETERINARY PRACTICES

As successful as Prolotherapy is for people, it is perhaps even more effective on animals. This may be largely due to the fact that animals eat better than humans do. Your pet rarely treats himself to a triple hot fudge banana brownie triple scoop topped with whipped cream and nuts, or spends more time in the potato chip aisle than the vegetable aisle of the grocery store.

Animals can and do experience pain, just like humans. The only difference is they cannot tell you they are in pain. Animals in pain may become listless, move constantly, groan, and whimper. If the pain is in a weight-bearing joint such as the hip, the animal will limp. The same causes of pain in humans generally apply to animals. As a matter of fact, we have learned most of what we know about pain and pain management in humans from animal studies. Tests on dogs, for example, have shown that hip joint laxity is the most important and reliable factor in determining the likelihood of degenerative joint disease of the hip.[1] A logical conclusion is that ligament laxity causes arthritis in dogs. I contend that this situation also occurs in humans. This is the physiological basis of why Prolotherapy stops the progression of the arthritic process. By strengthening the ligaments that surround the joints, Prolotherapy makes the joints stronger. Strong joints do not get arthritis, only loose or weak ones.

S. Fubini, D.V.M., stated that "lameness related to joint disorders has been reported to be a leading cause of disability among thoroughbred race horses."[2] Articular cartilage degeneration is the first sign of osteoarthritis in horses, a common irreversible joint disease. Experiments have clearly indicated that intra-articularly (inside the joint) administered steroids cause depletion of proteoglycan from articular cartilage in normal equine (horse) joints [3,4] and exacerbate osteoarthritic changes in diseased joints.[5,6] In other words, steroids cause the degeneration of the cartilage which leads to osteoarthritis. Steroids cause the same harmful effects in animals as they do in humans. Animals run from steroid injections, but humans will pay big bucks for them.

According to Dr. Fauley, "In traditional veterinary medicine, an animal's pain is typically treated with anti-inflammatory medicine and/or a steroid injection." These treatments do reduce the pain but very seldom cure it. "I believe Prolotherapy is a treatment modality that shows promise to have more definitive results on relieving pain in animals."[7]

Although anti-inflammatory medications and steroid injections reduce pain in animals, they do so at the cost of destroying tissue. In a study conducted by Siraya Chunekamrai, D.V.M., Ph.D., horses treated with eight weekly shots of a steroid commonly used in humans exhibited tremendously detrimental effects in the injected tissue. Some of the effects included chondrocyte necrosis (cartilage cell damage), hypocellularity (decreased number of cells) in the joint, decreased proteoglycan content and synthesis, and decreased collagen synthesis in the injected joint. All of these effects were permanent.

Chunekamrai concluded, "... the effects on cartilage of intra-articular injections of methylprednisolone acetate (a steroid) were not ameliorated at eight weeks after eight weekly injections, or sixteen weeks after a single injection. Cartilage remained bio-chemically and metabolically impaired."[8] In this study, some of the joints were injected only one time. Even after one steroid injection, cartilage remained bio-chemically and metabolically impaired. Other studies have confirmed similar harmful effects of steroids on joint and cartilage tissue.[9,10] A cortisone shot can permanently damage joints. Prolotherapy injections have the opposite effect—they permanently strengthen joints.

"Not just a few animals, I've treated hundreds," explains Michael Herron, D.V.M., an orthopedic animal specialist. "Our healing time of muscle, tendon, and ligament injuries has been accelerated by a third, just by using Sclerotherapy." Sclerotherapy is another name for Prolotherapy. "I've treated just about every muscle, ligament, and tendon in greyhound racers and found Sclerotherapy to be extremely effective. Most animals require only one treatment and quickly return to racing."[11]

Owners of Greyhound racers cannot afford to not let their dogs go back to racing so they turn to Prolotherapy. The question is: Why do athletes turn to cortisone shots and not to Prolotherapy? If the NFL, NBA, or PGA had a Prolotherapist on their medical staff, the athletes' time on injured reserve would significantly decrease.

Dr. Herron has used Sclerotherapy to effectively treat a partial Achilles tear in dogs. The most commonly treated area in a dog, however, is the wrist. Dr. Herron explained that dogs support 60 percent of their weight on the front paw wrist area. Therefore, this becomes the area where the ligaments require strengthening. Sclerotherapy is used anywhere in the animal where the ligaments are injured. Dr. Herron claims an 85 percent success rate in eliminating pain and disability with only

one Sclerotherapy treatment in the animals that he treats.[12]

SUMMARY

Prolotherapy, because it stimulates ligament and tendon growth, can be used anywhere a ligament or tendon is located. It does not matter if it is a dog, cat, horse, bull, parakeet, llama, or Johnny's pet gold fish. In the treatment of both chronic and acutely painful conditions in animals, Prolotherapy has been more than 85 percent successful with only one treatment. If utilized to its full extent, Prolotherapy can end most of the needless suffering of animals (and humans). It is for this reason many animal owners are choosing to Prolo their animal's pain away.

EPILOGUE

G ustav A. Hemwall, M.D., the world's most experienced Prolotherapist and my mentor, recently gave me the sad news of his retirement. I suppose after 60 years of practicing medicine and more than 40 years of giving four million Prolotherapy injections, he has the right.

His retirement reminds me of a passage in the Bible written by the apostle Paul: "I have fought the good fight, I have finished the race, I have kept the faith: Now there is in store for me the crown of righteousness, which the Lord, the righteous Judge, will award to me on that day—not only to me, but also to all who have longed for his appearing."[1]

It has been said that when a good thing ends another wonderful thing begins. I have been planning to write this book for years. The first draft was completed the week after Dr. Hemwall announced his retirement. People like K. Dean Reeves, M.D., Ed Magaziner, M.D., Rodney Van Pelt, M.D., Gerald Montgomery, M.D., Jeffery Patterson, D.O., Mark Wheaton, M.D., John Merriman, M.D., and I will carry on Dr. Hemwall's message. God is faithful, God loves us, and ultimately pain, as any trial, should lead us to Him. The needle is mightier than the knife. The ligament, not the nerve, is the cause of chronic pain. Correct diagnoses are made with the thumb, not the X-ray machine. **There is a cure for chronic pain. That cure is Prolotherapy.**

Nutrition and Chronic Pain

Congratulations! You have made it this far in the book. I hope you enjoyed it. Now you know why ligament and tendon weakness is commonly the cause of chronic pain and what can be done about it.

Prolotherapy starts the growth of ligament and tendon tissue, but *you* grow the tissue. If you stock your body with all the nutrients available—amino acids, vitamins, minerals, and essential fatty acids—optimum health and strong tissue will be the result.

Many people do not realize that a lunch salad does not provide them with three weeks worth of nutrition. I once asked a patient how many vegetable servings he consumed per day.

"Three," he replied.

I then asked him how he came to this conclusion.

"Well, for lunch I usually have a hamburger."

"So?" I exclaimed in my sophisticated English.

"There is ketchup, tomato, and onion on my hamburger. That's three."

I'm sorry to say, but condiments and hamburger toppings are not complete vegetable servings.

THE IMPORTANCE OF NUTRITION

Nutrients, like minerals and most vitamins, are water soluble. Consequently, whatever the body does not need for that day will be excreted in the urine. Therefore, vitamins and minerals need to be consumed daily to achieve optimum health. In their food pyramid, the United States government recommends consuming two to four servings of fruit and three to five servings of vegetables per day. The dietary habits of most Americans fall far short of meeting these recommendations.

During the past 40 years, the amount of nutrition in food products has declined largely due to poor soil quality. Today, it is very difficult to obtain adequate daily nutrients even when strictly adhering to the food pyramid. Manure is no longer used as fertilizer and the land is never given a chance to rest. An apple today does not have the same nutrient value apples did 40 years ago. Organic apples fertilized with manure are more nutritious than apples grown with chemical fertilizers and sprayed with pesticides. I am a strong advocate of organic foods. Besides their nutritional value, organically grown foods do not contain the chemical toxins found in conventionally grown foods.

Vitamins and mineral supplements, especially a general multivitamin, will aid you in your quest to obtain enough daily nutrients. Other specific nutrients may be helpful, depending on your health. If you seek preventative care from a Natural Medicine physician and develop an interest in nutrition, you will soon be on the road to wellness. (*See Appendix C, Natural Medicine Resources, for organizations that provide referrals for Natural Medicine physicians.*)

A SUPPLEMENT TO PROMOTE HEALING

People getting Prolotherapy treatments often ask me if there are supplements they should take to aid in the healing of their ligaments and tendons. The first step would be to undergo Metabolic Typing to determine what foods will contribute to the healing process. The next step would be to take a good general vitamin and mineral supplement. (*See Appendix C, Natural Medicine Resources, for nutritional companies and supplements I recommend.*)

I recommend a supplement that I formulated for Orthomolecular Products that is specifically designed to help grow ligament and tendon tissue. The product, called Ortho Prolo Max, has unique ingredients that have been shown to help collagen formation in the body. Ortho Prolo Max contains the following ingredients:

Ingredients	Reason for ingredient being in the product
L-Proline	Collagen is one-third Proline
L-Cysteine	Critical to soft tissue healing
Grape Seed Procyanadins	Natural antioxidant
Glucosamine Sulfate	A component of tendon and ligament tissue
Horsetail herb	Natural source of silica
RNA	Help fibroblasts (which grow collagen) replicate
Centella Asiatica Herb	Enhances connective tissue structure
MSM (Methylsulfonylmethane)	Natural source of sulfur

The product also contains other ingredients that I believe help soft tissue heal, thereby aiding Prolotherapy treatments.

Lastly, specific nutrients may be added depending on an individual's needs. If someone appears to be tired, I may add Ginseng, Licoric Root, or other nutrients for adrenal support. If muscle spasms are a major issue then more magnesium, calcium, or potassium may be added. The Metabolic Typing will also give some indication that other nutrients are needed. Don't wait until you are sick. Prevent sickness by paying attention to your health now.

METABOLIC TYPING

At my Natural Medicine clinic in Oak Park, Illinois, I use a laboratory test called Metabolic Typing to determine specific nutritional needs. Metabolic Typing is a process that determines a person's basic underlying physiology. In simplistic terms, some people have the physiology of a lion and others have that of a giraffe. No, it does not mean some people are hairy and others have long necks. A lion survives best on a high protein diet, whereas a giraffe fares better on a vegetarian-based diet. Metabolic Typing can determine which type of nutritional program best suits a particular individual and what vitamins and minerals are needed.

Metabolic Typing involves monitoring a patient's detailed diet history with subsequent general well-being after they eat various foods. Lion metabolic types tend to feel better after eating meat, chicken, fish, and other foods high in protein. Giraffe metabolic types feel better after consuming salad, fruit, vegetables, pasta, coffee, and tea.

Lions generally have acid blood, alkaline urine, and are called acid blood types. Giraffes generally have alkaline blood, acid urine, and are called alkaline blood types. The acid-alkaline terminology refers to the pH of the various body fluids. Acid pH means the pH is lower than normal, whereas alkaline pH means the pH is higher than normal.

In order to determine a metabolic type, the patient provides urine, saliva, and blood samples after having fasted for 15 hours and at one-and-a-half hours after eating a meal. The pH of each fluid is tested. Other tests are done on the urine sample to provide a "metabolic picture" of the patient's body functions, as described by Carey Reams, Ph.D.[1] The patient is then given a 50-gram glucose fruit drink and fingerstick blood sugars are taken every 30 minutes for a total of 90 minutes to determine how quickly the body metabolizes food. Some people utilize food quickly and are known as fast oxidizers. Those who use food slowly are called slow oxidizers. People are then divided into several categories, depending on whether they are acid, alkaline, or balanced blood types and whether they are fast, slow, or balanced oxidizers.

The classic lion is a fast oxidizer, acid blood type. This person feels great eating meat and other foods high in protein. Since the lion is a fast oxidizer, it needs food that is utilized by the body slowly. Fat and protein require lengthy digestion before becoming available to the body to use as an energy source. These patients require a high protein, higher fat, low carbohydrate diet, as well as various supplements and vitamins that balance the pH. Vitamin E, vitamin B-3, B-12, B-5, fish oils, zinc, iodine, and calcium will aid in this process. Items such as vitamin C in the form of ascorbic acid are very acidic and are therefore excluded.

The classic giraffe is a slow oxidizer, alkaline blood type. Because the giraffe utilizes food slowly, it needs food that is easily absorbed like fruits and vegetables. The giraffe feels best eating a vegetarian-based diet and requires less protein than the lion. Supplements to balance a giraffe's pH include alfalfa or wheat grass, vitamins and minerals like vitamin C, vitamins B-1, B-2, B-3, B-6, magnesium, chromium, and potassium may be recommended.

Metabolic Typing helps explain why some patients maintain good health eating a vegetarian diet and why others can do the same eating a high protein diet. There is no one diet that is the best for everyone. Contrary to popular belief, patients can lose weight and lower their cholesterol while consuming a diet high in protein and fat. When was the last time you saw a fat lion? Lion types have trouble with obesity and heart disease when they eat a diet high in carbohydrates. Lion types need to eat less refined carbohydrates like white bread, pasta, potatoes, and food high in sugar.

Opposites do attract. A lion metabolic type usually marries a giraffe metabolic type. My wife, Marion, is pure giraffe. She even has the neck! She eats a vegetarian-based diet. If she eats too much fat during a meal, she has immediate bloating and feels terrible. I am a pure lion. A pizza will put me to sleep, but a juicy hamburger makes me feel great. Do I have a cholesterol problem? No. My cholesterol is below normal.

Another aspect of determining the proper foods for a person involves checking blood type. Depending on a person's blood type, certain foods are better than others. Peter D'Adamo, M.D., has written a comprehensive book on this subject titled *Eat Right for Your Type*.[2]

Remember there is no one diet for everyone. Each person requires a diet and supplement program for their body type. To learn more about Metabolic Typing, read *Biobalance*, by Rudolf Wiley, Ph.D.[3]

I learned about Metabolic Typing and Reams testing from wonderful clinicians, Gail Gelsinger, R.N., Harold Kristal, D.D.S., Mike and Sue Aberle, and Gary Martin, Ph.D. Anyone wanting to undergo Metabolic Typing should contact my wife, Marion, or one of the other clinicians listed below:

Gary Martin, Ph.D.
Biological Immunity Research Institute
13610 N. Scottsdale Rd., Suite 14
Scottsdale, AZ 85254-4056
(800) 294-6686

Marion A. Hauser, M.S., R.D.
Caring Medical & Rehabilitation Services, S.C.
715 Lake St., Suite 600
Oak Park, IL 60301
(708) 848-7789
(708) 848-7763 fax

Gail Gelsinger, R.N.
Cornerstone to Health
P.O. Box 233
Robesonia, PA 19551
(610) 693-6086
(610) 693-5858 fax

Harold J. Kristal, D.D.S.
Nutritional Dentistry
520 Tamalpais Drive, Suite 205
Corte Madera, CA 94925
(415) 924-2571

Mike and Sue Aberle
Promise Outreach
R.R. 2, P.O. Box 61
Cashton, WI 54619
(608) 634-2440

Neural Therapy

S ome people experience chronic pain that is not due to ligament or tendon weakness. Some chronic pain stems from nerve irritation. This type of pain may be relieved by a treatment known as Neural Therapy.

Neural Therapy is a gentle healing technique developed in Germany that involves the injection of local anesthetics into autonomic ganglia, peripheral nerves, scars, glands, acupuncture points, trigger points, and other tissues.[1] What are autonomic ganglia? The body contains two nervous systems: the somatic and the autonomic. The somatic nervous system is under a person's voluntary control. The autonomic nervous system functions automatically. The autonomic ganglia is the place where the center of the autonomic nerves are located.

SOMATIC AND AUTONOMIC NERVOUS SYSTEMS

The nerves in the somatic nervous system control skin sensation and muscle movement. Picking up a cup of tea, for example, requires the somatic nervous system to sense the cup with the fingers and contract the muscles to lift the cup. These are the same nerves that are pinched in a herniated disc.

The autonomic nervous system is automatically activated. Life-sustaining functions like breathing, blood flow, pupil dilation, and perspiration are activated by the autonomic nervous system. People do not think about the blood vessels in their hands constricting when they are outside on a cold, winter day. This occurs automatically. The functioning of the autonomic nervous system is crucial as it controls blood flow throughout the body. Illness often begins when the blood flow to an extremity or an organ is decreased.

A limb with decreased blood flow feels cold and may experience dull burning pain. Even atrophy (breakdown) of the skin and muscles may occur. Decreased blood flow to an organ hinders its ability to function. Decreased blood flow to the thyroid gland may result in hypothyroidism. In this instance, the amount of thyroid hormone the body produces is decreased, resulting in sluggishness, weight gain, and lower body temperature. Does that sound like anyone you know?

Disturbed autonomic nervous system function has been implicated in the following diseases: headaches, migraines, dizziness, confusion, optic neuritis, chronic ear infections, tinnitus, vertigo, hay fever, sinusitis, tonsillitis, asthma, liver disease, gallbladder disease, menstrual pain, eczema, and a host of others.[2] Neural Therapy, because it increases blood flow, may have profoundly positive effects on such conditions.

INTERFERENCE FIELDS

The founder of Neural Therapy, Ferdinand Huneke, M.D., felt one of its beneficial effects was the elimination of interference fields. An interference field is any pathologically damaged tissue, which on account of an excessively strong or long-standing stimulus or of a summation of stimuli that cannot be abated, is in a state of unphysiological permanent excitation.[3] In layman's terms, any time a tissue is injured it can continually excite the autonomic nervous system. These centers of irritation through the autonomic nervous system may cause disease in other parts of the body.

Most interference fields are found in the head region. According to Dr. Huneke, teeth and tonsils are the two most common probably because they are close to the brain and nerves. An infected tooth can set up an interference field causing a person to have chronic low back pain or a heart arrhythmia. A patient may have chronic low back pain that is unresponsive to surgical and conservative treatments because an interference field is present.

Scars are the next most common interference fields. Any scar, no matter how small or old, even if it dates back to early childhood, can be the interference field causing therapy-resistant rheumatoid arthritis, hearing loss, sciatica, or other serious disorders.[4]

A good analogy of the interference field is heart arrhythmia, or irregular heart beats. In a heart arrhythmia an area of the heart sends off an independent, electrical impulse. This impulse is not under the normal control of the heart's electrical system. It acts independently and automatically. During a heart attack, the heart may produce extra beats, called premature ventricular contractions (PVCs). One of the standard treatments for PVCs is an intravenous infusion of Lidocaine, an anesthetic. This treatment effectively stops this type of arrhythmia.

NEURAL THERAPY AS PAIN MANAGEMENT

Neural Therapy involves the injection of anesthetic solutions, such as Lidocaine or procaine, into these interference fields. The areas injected may include various areas of the teeth, tonsils, autonomic nervous system nerves, or ganglia, somatic or peripheral nerves, scars, or the area surrounding various organs. Immediate pain relief is often observed after the first injection because nerve irritation has been resolved.

Most traditional physicians are not aware of the role of the autonomic nervous system or do not diagnose problems involving it because an autonomic nervous system cannot be tested. The autonomic nervous system does not appear on X-rays; only somatic nervous system nerves can be seen.

To diagnose an autonomic nervous system problem, the clinician must understand interference fields as well as Neural Therapy. An autonomic nervous system disorder should be suspected if any of the following conditions are evident: burning pain, excessively cool or hot extremities, pale or red hands or feet, skin sensitivity to touch, scars, root canals, chronic problems occurring after an infection or accident, chronic pain not responsive to other forms of therapy, shooting burning nerve pain, pinched nerve, or a chronic medical condition that has not responded to other treatments.

Neural Therapy is used more frequently as a healing modality in European countries than in the United States. To find an experienced Neural Therapist, contact the American Association of Neural Therapy, 4100 S. W. Edmunds, Suite 101, Seattle, WA 98116. (888) NEURAL-K or (888) 638-7255.

To learn more about Neural Therapy, consult the *Illustrated Atlas of the Techniques of Neural Therapy with Local Anesthetics*, a textbook from Germany.[5] The American Association of Neural Therapy also offers courses under the guidance of Dietrich K. Klinghardt, M.D., Ph.D.

At my office, Neural Therapy has been a wonderful, adjunctive therapy for the treatment of chronic pain and illness. A person with chronic pain often has evidence of both ligament laxity and autonomic nervous system dysfunction. In such a case, both Prolotherapy and Neural Therapy are warranted. Because chronic pain sometimes has an autonomic nervous system component, many are choosing to Neural Therapy their pain away!

Natural Medicine Resources

M any people suffer from pain partially because their bodies have lost the ability to heal soft tissue injuries completely. If someone receives Prolotherapy for a weakened ligament or tendon, but their body lacks a vital nutrient, healing can still be incomplete. It is important to consume all vital nutrients each day to assist soft tissue healing.

The following are companies and products I use and recommend:

Kylea Health and Nutrition
P.O. Box 399
Glen Ellyn, IL 60138
(888) 557-5700
Kylea Health and Nutrition has superb nutritional products that have the endorsement of James Balch, M.D., author of the national best-seller Prescription for Nutritional Healing. *Also, what I like about the company is that the owner, Joseph Costello commits 10 percent of the proceeds to worthy charitable causes.*

Metabolic Management
16180 E. 12000 N Rd.
Grant Park, IL 60940
(800) 373-1373
Joseph Buishas, the owner of Metabolic Management, has been in the nutrition business for many years. His company offers an array of herbs to help specific conditions. Their product called Thyrostim, for example, contains kelp and other nutrients that help patients who appear to have symptoms of hypothyroidism. Their glandular products and enzymes including bromelain are excellent. I appreciate the support Metabolic Management has given to Beulah Land Natural Medicine Clinic.

Orthomolecular Products
2771 Cedar Drive
Plover, WI 54467
(800) 332-2351
I use Ortho Prolo Max, which I developed for Orthomolecular Products, specifically for people who have a soft tissue injury. Ortho Prolo Max has been helpful in assisting healing in all the conditions discussed in this book including fibromyalgia, arthritis, and chronic pain. The product contains bioflavenoids, natural cartilage, amino acids, natural silica, nucleic acids, as well as various minerals and herbs to assist healing. (See Appendix A, Nutrition and Chronic Pain.) Orthomolecular Products, owned by Gary Powers, also has some of the best products for fighting infections including colds, worms, parasites, and yeast.

Shaklee Vitamins/Herbs
(800) 372-0050
Take Vita-Lea 4/day and B-complex 4/day as a multiple vitamin/mineral supplement. If getting enough protein is an issue, take Shaklee protein powders. To obtain more information about Shaklee Vitamins/Herbs, or to order products, call Marjorie Felton Petry at (800) 372-0050. Marjorie is very knowledgeable when it comes to vitamins and good health. She loves to educate people and enjoys getting calls.

Organizations that provide referral lists of doctors who utilize natural treatments:

American Academy of Anti-Aging Medicine
1341 W. Fullerton, Suite 111
Chicago, IL 60614
(773) 528-4333
(773) 528-5390 fax

American College for Advancement in Medicine
23121 Verdugo Drive, Suite 204
Laguna Hills, CA 92653
(800) 532-3688

American Holistic Medical Association
4101 Lake Boone Trail, Suite 201
Raleigh, NC 27607
(919) 787-5181

American Preventive Medicine Association
459 Walker Rd.
Great Falls, VA 22066
(800) 230-2762
(703) 759-6711 fax

International Bio-Oxidative Medicine
Foundation
P.O. Box 891954
Oklahoma City, OK 73189
(405) 478-4266

The Rheumatoid Disease Foundation
5106 Old Harding Rd.
Franklin, TN 37064-9400
(615) 646-1030

Journals and newsletters that provide information on Natural Medicine:

Alternative Medicine Digest
21 ½ Main St.
Tiburon, CA 94920
(415) 789-8700
(800) 546-6707 (Subscription only)

Alternatives
Dr. David Williams
Phillips Publishing International, Inc.
7811 Montrose Rd.
Potomac, MD 20854
(301) 340-2100

Clinical Pearls News
IT Services
3301 Alta Arden #2
Sacramento, CA 95825
(916) 483-1085
(916) 483-1431 fax

Health & Healing Newsletter
Julian Whitaker, M.D.
Phillips Publishing International, Inc.
7811 Montrose Rd.
Potomac, MD 20854
(301) 340-2100

Nutrition & Healing
Alan Gaby, M.D.
Jonathan Wright, M.D.
P.O. Box 84909
Phoenix, AZ 85071
(800) 528-0559
(602) 943-2363 fax

Second Opinion
William Campbell Douglass, M.D.
Second Opinion Publishing, Inc.
7100 Peachtree
Dunwoody, GA 30328
(800) 728-2288

Townsend Letter for Doctors & Patients
911 Tyler St.
Port Townsend, WA 98368
(360) 385-6021

For information about a specific Natural Medicine topic, contact:

A. Keith Brewer International Science Library
325 North Central Ave.
Richland, WI 53581
(608) 647-6513
The library and its staff provide a wealth of knowledge on any health care topic. They will provide anyone with written information on health-related questions. If I am unable to answer a question concerning one of my patients, I consult the staff and resources at this library.

Prolotherapy Referral List

W hile Prolotherapy is a technique that is still relatively unknown, it is gaining popularity. In this appendix, I have included a list of physicians in the United States and Canada who utilize Prolotherapy in their practice for the treatment of chronic pain. I have also included information on books that have been published on the subject.

Physicians mentioned in this book who utilize the Hackett technique of Prolotherapy:

Dr. James Cade
Prolotherapy Pain Clinic
6737 Highway 98 West
Hattiesburg, MS 39402
(601) 261-0074

Ross A. Hauser, M.D.
Caring Medical & Rehabilitation Services, S.C.
715 Lake St., Suite 600
Oak Park, IL 60301
(708) 848-7789
(708) 848-7763 fax

Gustav A. Hemwall, M.D.
715 Lake St., Suite 605
Oak Park, IL 60301
(708) 848-7773

Bernadette Goheen Kohn, D.O.
4309 Medical Center Drive
Suite B-201
McHenry, IL 60050
(815) 344-7951
(815) 344-0076 fax

Ed Magaziner, M.D.
1323 Route 27
Summerset, NJ 08873
(908) 220-6600

John Merriman, M.D.
2325 S. Harvard Ave., Suite 308
Tulsa, OK 74114
(918) 744-5959

Jean Paul Ouellette, M.D.
2555 St. Joseph Blvd., Suite 206
Orleans, Ontario
Canada, K1C 156
(613) 824-4223
(613) 824-2418 fax

K. Dean Reeves, M.D.
155 S. 18th Street, Suite 180
Kansas City, KS 66102
(913) 321-0033

Rodney Van Pelt, M.D.
665 N. State St.
Ukiah, CA 95482
(707) 463-1782

Other physicians personally known by the author who utilize the Hackett technique of Prolotherapy:

Michael J. Adams, D.O.
7 Hamilton Lane
St. Peters, MO 63376
(314) 397-5757

Fred Cenaiko, M.D.
Wakaw Hospital
Box 309
Wakaw, Saskatchewan
Canada, S0K 4P0
(306) 233-4611
(306) 233-4641

John Finkenstadt, M.D.
North Syracuse Health Center
792 N. Main St.
North Syracuse, NY 13212
(315) 458-6852

Gerardo Cajero Callejas
Av. Villado 120
Toluco, Mexico
(011) 52-72-15-25-74

Michael Jacobson, D.O.
9771 Otterbein Rd.
Cincinnati, OH 45241
(513) 563-9909

George Kramer, M.D.
PDR
903 1st Street North
Hopkins, MN 55543
(612) 931-3999

Thomas Masten, M.D.
550 Harrison Center, Suite 130
Syracuse, NY 13200
(315) 472-2225

Bernard Milton, M.D.
Braidwood Medical Center
233 East Reed St.
Braidwood, IL 60408
(815) 458-6700

Gerald Montgomery, M.D.
222 Summitt Spring Rd.
Poland Spring, ME 04274
(207) 998-2034

Jeffrey Patterson, D.O.
University of Wisconsin Medical Center
Department of Family Medicine
777 S. Mills St.
Madison, WI 53715
(608) 241-9020

John Pletincks, M.D.
Maranatha Pain Clinic
6314 Whiskey Creek Drive
Fort Meyers, FL 33919
(941) 433-1221

Samuel Schwartz, D.O.
1822 West Indian School Rd.
Phoenix, AZ 85015-5206
(602) 277-8911

Timothy Speciale, D.O.
495 Delaware St., Suite 2
Tonawanda, NY 14150
(716) 692-2723
(716) 692-5173 fax

William Tham, M.D.
706 Giddings Ave., Suite 2-B
Annapolis, MD 21401
(410) 268-2943

Mark T. Wheaton, M.D.
Ridgehill Professional Building
2000 Plymouth Rd., Suite 175
Minnetonka, MN 55305
(612) 593-0500
(612) 593-0303 fax

A list of physicians who utilize Prolotherapy but not necessarily the Hackett technique can be obtained from:

American Association of Orthopedic Medicine
90 S. Cascade Ave., Suite 1190
Colorado Springs, CO 80909
(800) 992-2063

American College of Osteopathic Pain Management and Sclerotherapy (ACOPMS)
107 Maple Ave., Silverside Heights
Wilmington, DE 19809
(302) 792-9280

Physicians desiring training in Prolotherapy can contact the two organizations listed above as well as:

George S. Hackett Foundation
c/o Gustav A. Hemwall, M.D.
715 Lake St., Suite 605
Oak Park, IL 60301
(708) 848-7773

Courses are held each October. The author believes this is the best course on Prolotherapy. A mission trip doing Prolotherapy in Honduras is held each spring.

Marion A. Hauser, M.S., R.D.
Caring Medical & Rehabilitation Services, S.C.
715 Lake St., Suite 600
Oak Park, IL 60301
(708) 848-7789
(708) 848-7763 fax
We run a charity clinic in southern Illinois where a Prolotherapy seminar is held each year. This is an excellent place to get hands-on Prolotherapy experience.

Thomas Dorman, M.D.
Tacoma Clinic
515 W. Harrison St., Suite 200
Kent, WA 98032
(206) 854-4900
(206) 859-8660 fax
Dr. Dorman knows virtually everything there is to know about Prolotherapy and is a prolific writer on the subject. He also teaches several courses.

William Faber, D.O.
Milwaukee Pain Clinic
6529 West Fon du Lac Ave.
Milwaukee, WI 53218
(414) 464-7246
Dr. Faber has written several books on Prolotherapy and offers individualized teaching on reconstructive therapy.

Veterinarians who administer Prolotherapy:

Shaun Fauley, D.V.M.
Care Animal Clinic
531 West 87th St.
Naperville, IL 60565
(630) 355-6164

Michael Herron, D.V.M.
Department of Small Animal Medicine
College of Veterinary Medicine & Surgery
Texas A&M University
College Station, TX 77843-4474
(409) 845-2351

Other Prolotherapy resources:

Teaching Tapes
Teaching tapes that illustrate the technique of Prolotherapy by David Brewer, M.D., Ross Hauser, M.D., Gustav A. Hemwall, M.D., and Jean-Paul Ouellette, M.D., can be ordered by calling (708) 848-7789.

List of Doctors
For a complete list of doctors who have learned the technique of Prolotherapy at a Hackett foundation meeting, send $5 and a self-addressed stamped envelope to: Caring Medical & Rehabilitation Services, S.C., 715 Lake St., Suite 600, Oak Park, IL 60301.

List of Patients
If you would like to speak with someone who has had Prolotherapy for a condition similar to yours, send a self-addressed, stamped envelope and $5 to: Caring Medical and Rehabilitation Services, S.C., 715 Lake St., Oak Park, IL 60301. We will send you a list of patients to contact.

Books
Ligament and Tendon Relaxation Treated by Prolotherapy, by George S. Hackett, M.D., Gustav A. Hemwall, M.D., and Gerald Montgomery, M.D., can be ordered from the Institute in Basic Life Principles, Box One, Oak Brook, IL 60522-3001. (630) 323-9800 (extension 740). Ask for basic care publication department. This is the updated version of the original book by Dr. Hackett and is the best book to date on Prolotherapy.

Diagnosis and Injection Techniques in Orthopaedic Medicine, by Thomas Dorman, M.D., can be ordered from Williams & Wilkins, 428 E. Preston St., Baltimore, MD 21202. (410) 528-4000.

Pain Pain Go Away and *Instant Pain Relief*, by William J. Faber, D.O., and Morton Walker, D.P.M. To order, call Dr. Faber's office at (404) 464-7246. Or write to him at 6529 West Fon du Lac Ave., Milwaukee, WI 53218. Or, contact Freelance Communications at (203) 322-1551. Or, write to Freelance Communications at 484 High Ridge Rd., Stamford, CT 06905-3020.

APPENDIX E

George S. Hackett AMA Presentations

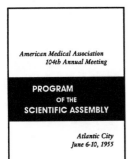

American Medical Association
104th Annual Meeting
Program of the Scientific Assembly
Atlantic City, June 6-10, 1955

Diagnosis and Treatment of Back Disabilities.
George S. Hackett, Canton, Ohio.

"Relaxation of the posterior ligaments of the spine and pelvis is the most frequent cause of back pain and disability. Diagnosis is made by trigger point pressure and confirmed by injecting an anaesthetic within the ligament. The local and referred pain are immediately reproduced and disappear within two minutes. The patient's confidence is established. Treatment consists of injection of a proliferant within the ligament which stimulates the production of bone and fibrous tissue, which becomes permanent. New areas of referred pain in the groin, buttock, and extremities have been identified during the past 16 years while making over 3,000 injections within the ligaments of 563 patients, with 82% considering themselves cured. Ages range from 15 to 81 years. Longest duration before treatment was 49 years; the average was 4 ½ years. X-rays of animal experiments carried out over two years reveal the proliferation of abundant permanent tissue at the fibro-osseous junction."

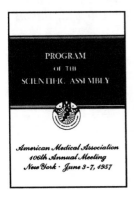

American Medical Association
106th Annual Meeting
Program of the Scientific Assembly
New York, June 3-7, 1957

Pain, Referred Pain and Sciatica in Back Diagnosis and Treatment.
George S. Hackett, Mercy Hospital, Canton, Ohio.

"Referred pain into the extremities and sciatica results more often from relaxed ligaments of unstable joints than from all other causes combined. Referred pain areas into the groin, lower abdomen, genitalia, buttock and extremities to as far as the toes from articular ligaments that support the lumbar and pelvic joints have been established from observations while making over 10,000 intraligamentous injections in the diagnosis and treatment of 1,207 patients during the past 18 years. Articular ligament relaxation has been found to be the cause of more chronic low back disability than from any other entity. The trigger points of pain of specific disabled ligaments have been established. In diagnosis, knowledge of the referred pain areas directs attention to specific ligaments, and in conjunction with the trigger points of pain, enables the physician to accurately locate the cause of the disability. Ninety percent of the patients with joint instability are cured by the intraligamentous injection of a proliferating solution which stimulates the production of new bone and fibrous tissue cells to permanently strengthen the ligaments."

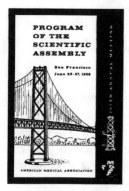

American Medical Association
107th Annual Meeting
Program of the Scientific Assembly
San Francisco, June 23-27, 1958

Cervical Whiplash Injury.
George S. Hackett, Canton, Ohio.

"Chronic whiplash cervical pain has its origin within incompetent occipital tendons and cervical articular ligaments which stretch under normal tension and permit an overstimulation of the nonstretchable sensory nerve fibrils at the fibro-osseous junction. It results in headache and specific referred pain areas to as far as the eyes, temples, and fingers. The diagnosis is invariably confirmed by intraligamentous needling with an anesthetic solution. 82% of 1656 patients throughout 19 years considered themselves permanently cured by Prolotherapy (rehabilitation of an incompetent structure by the proliferation of new cells—bone and fibrous tissue "weld")."

The information in this appendix is from abstracts of Dr. Hackett's presentations and is used with permission of the American Medical Association, Chicago, Illinois.

Insurance Reimbursement Letters

When the issue of the efficacy of Prolotherapy found its way to the courts in Canada for the first time last year (where socialized medicine reigns and governmental bodies do not want to pay for certain medical procedures) for lumbar disc syndrome, the verdict read "on the basis of all the evidence, the Prolotherapy treatment administered to the patient was and is a safe and efficacious treatment."[1]

Similar cases have been noted in the United States. When an insurer in the state of Washington did not pay for the Prolotherapy treatment that relieved a person's chronic low back pain, the case was brought to trial. The Washington State Health Care Authority found that the Sclerotherapy (Prolotherapy) treatments the patient received for back pain were "medically necessary."

The Washington State Heath Care Authority also ruled that the treatments needed to be paid by the insurer. This judgement was made June 8, 1992 by Margaret T. Stanley, Administrator, Washington State Health Care, in the case of Joel M. Greene vs. Uniform Medical Plan.[2]

In the following pages, I have provided copies of letters from the Chicago Medical Society (one of the largest branches of the American Medical Association) and insurance carriers regarding reimbursement for Prolotherapy. Please note on three separate occasions, the Medical Practice Committee of the Chicago Medical Society found Prolotherapy to be an accepted procedure that deserved reimbursement by the insurance carrier.

Realize that insurance companies hold the right whether or not to reimburse for a specific therapy. The attached letters are for individual patients and reimbursement decisions were made on a case by case basis. All names and personal information have been withheld to respect the privacy of the individuals.

Chicago
Medical Society
The Medical Society of Cook County

310 SOUTH MICHIGAN AVENUE, CHICAGO, ILLINOIS 60604. TELEPHONE (312) 922-0417

April 20, 1976

Gustav Hemwall, M.D.
715 Lake Street
Oak Park, IL   60301

Re:
Carrier: Aetna Life & Casualty
Date of Treatment: August 10, 1975
CMS No. 76-M-005

Dear Doctor Hemwall:

In response to the insurance carrier's request of whether your treatment is an approved and appropriate method, the Subcommittee on Insurance Mediation has made a decision on the above entitled matter.

On the basis of the information presented, it the Committee's opinion that this procedure is an accepted procedure.

By copy of this letter, the insurance carrier will be informed of our recommendation.

Cordially,

Carell Hutchinson, JR., M.D.
Chairman
Subcommittee on Insurance Mediation

CH:scm
cc: Aetna Life & Casualty

Chicago
Medical Society

The Medical Society of Cook County

810 South Michigan Avenue, Chicago, Illinois 60604. Telephone (312) 922-0417

November 1, 1979

Miss Karen M. Heckinger
Legal Research Assistant
Life Investors Insurance
    Company of America.
814 Commerce Drive
Oak Brook, IL   60521

Re: CMS File 79-G-069

Your File
    Policy No. F-9-3888
    National Ass'n. Business Owners

Dear Miss Heckinger:

After extensive inquiries by the Medical Practice Committee
on the efficacy and the legitimacy of the treatment referred
to as 'prolotherapy' we are left with the conclusion that
there is no body of scientific data which supports this method of medical treatment. While we are unable to state that
the treament is effective and accepted by the medical community, neither can we state that it is rejected by the medical community since we do not have scientific data upon which
to base our judgment.

It is the opinion of the Committee that, while the treatment
does not enjoy widespread acceptance in medical circles, it is
a well recognized procedure in veterinary medicine: animal
models of disease and treatment form the basis for a great deal
of medical knowledge and progress.

It is significant to this Committee that Dr. Hemwall has performed this procedure on a great many people over an eighteen
year period of time and our Society has never received a patient complaint on the procedure. It appears to us that this

page two   CMS File 79-G-069

record speaks for successful treatment. We do not feel that
either we, or an insurance carrier, are in a position to declare an uncommon, but apparently successful, procedure as an
improper one. Because the method is not widely used does not
mean that it is not compensable.

A search of our records reveals that another Committee of our
Society was presented with a similar question regarding 'prolotherapy' and they found it an accepted procedure and recommended payment of the physician's fees. We agree.

                          Sincerely,

                          Michael Treister, M.D.
                          Chairman
                          Medical Practice Committee

MT:WDF/SFO:vvm

xc: Gustav A. Hemwall, M.D.
    Edward J. King, Counsel

November 5, 1987

RE: Prolotherapy
Chubb Life America Insurance Co.

Group Policy No. 314295
Claim No. 725514

Dear

We apologize for the length of time this review has taken, however the Medical Practice Committee of the Chicago Medical Society has spent much time reviewing the subject of Prolotherapy. Attached is a copy of an article published in The Western Journal of Medicine, 1982, which is a study that attempts to establish the value of Prolotherapy. In addition, we have enclosed a list of references that address the use of this procedure.

The term Prolotherapy has not found favor with many insurance companies because it does not fit with their various codes. However, upon reviewing a list of procedures that have HCFA assigned codes published by Blue Shield of Illinois (HCSC) 5/15/86, Prolotherapy is coded M0076 on page 84. It is our understanding that two years ago, the Prolotherapy Association was incorporated into a new organization called the American Association of Orthopaedic Medicine. The insurance company may wish to contact this association for additional scientific studies.

We understand that this procedure has been used by many medical and osteopathic physicians both in this country and in Europe. It is significant that Dr. Hemwall has performed this procedure on many people for almost 30 years and our Society has never received a complaint on the use of the procedure. It appears to the committee that this record speaks for successful treatment, and it is long past the stage where it is considered experimental. It is our opinion that an insurance carrier is not in a position to declare a method that is not widely used, but apparently successful, an improper one.

Page - 2

In light of our current review, it is the opinion of the Medical Practice Committee that the procedure of ligament injection, known as Prolotherapy, is a clinically accepted procedure and we recommend payment of the physicians fees by the insurance company.

We thank you for bringing your concerns to our attention and by copy of this letter and attached materials, Chubb LifeAmerica Insurance Company will be informed of our recommendation.

Sincerely,

Peter C. Pulos, M.D.
Chairman
Medical Practice Committee

PCP:lm
cc: Steven Prylak
    Assistant Vice President
    Group Claims Department
    Chubb LifeAmerica

encls.

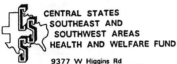

**CENTRAL STATES
SOUTHEAST AND
SOUTHWEST AREAS
HEALTH AND WELFARE FUND**

9377 W Higgins Rd
Rosemont IL 60018-4938
(800) 323-5000

April 23, 1996

ROSS A HAUSER MD
715 LAKE ST SUITE 600
OAK PARK   IL 60301

RE:

Dear Dr. Hauser :

This letter is in reply to your recent inquiry regarding
          need for prolotherapy treatments.

I am happy to say that the prolotherapy treatments will be payable
for four sessions one month apart from each other under the Major
Medical portion of Benefit Plan ET1. Under this Plan, there is a
$100 per calendar year deductible ($200 for the family). Once that
has been met, we will pay 80% of our reasonable and customary
allowance for all remaining eligible charges.   must be
covered on the date(s) on which services are rendered.

If you have any questions, please write the   Research   and
Correspondence Department at P.O. Box 5111, Des Plaines, IL 60017.

Sincerely,

Aileen M. Trola
Analyst
Research & Correspondence Dept.

cc:
cc: Local Union No. 706

M M A

Mennonite Mutual Aid
1110 North Main Street
Post Office Box 483
Goshen, IN 46527

Toll-free 1-800-348-7468
Telephone 219 533-9511
Fax 219 533-5264

June 17, 1997

Ross A. Hauser, M.D.
Caring Medical & Rehab Services, Inc.
715 Lake Street, Ste 600
Oak Park, IL 60301

Insured:
Patient: Agreement No.: 5090476
Effective Date: February 1, 1990

Thank you for inquiring about   's benefits for Prolotherapy. Our
medical review team has reviewed the packet of information you sent.

We will approve coverage for up to three treatments. After the $1,000 is
met, we will pay 80 percent of the next $5,000, then 100 percent to the end
of the calendar year. The maximum lifetime benefit is $1 million. The
deductible and coinsurance are applied each calendar year.

Benefits are limited to the reasonable and customary charges and the medical
team will review for proper coding.

A final decision on any claim cannot be made until we receive the actual
charges and review them according to the guidelines of the certificate.

Thank you for contacting us to verify the benefits. If you have further
questions about coverage we provide, please let me know.

Sincerely,

Polly Kauffman
Polly Kauffman
Managed Care Assistant

cc:

Beulah Land Natural Medicine Clinic

Beulah Land Natural Medicine Clinic is a charity clinic devoted through the grace of God to the prevention and treatment of human disease. This is accomplished through prayer, faithfulness to God through Jesus Christ, rest, nutrition, exercise, and the utilization of natural substances for healing and wellness.

Beulah Land Natural Medicine Clinic is located in very rural and very southern Illinois in the town of Thebes. Thebes is located one hour north of Paducah, Kentucky; one hour south of Carbondale, Illinois; and 30 minutes west of Cape Girardeau, Missouri. My wife, Marion, and I started the clinic in 1993.

Why would a Chicago couple choose Thebes, Illinois to start a charity Natural Medicine clinic? Good question. In 1985, Marion and I dedicated our lives to what we felt was the most important thing in life: faith in God through Jesus Christ. We both realized that where we go after this earthly life is more important than anything we have in this earthly life because life is finite, whereas eternity lasts forever.

At that time, we both came to realize what the Bible said was true. The Bible speaks about heaven in Revelation 21:27 saying, "Nothing impure will ever enter it, nor will anyone who does what is shameful or deceitful, but only those whose names were written in the Lamb's book of life."[1] We realized that we needed our names to be written in the Book of Life.

To have eternal life with God in heaven, we needed to accept Jesus Christ as our Savior. We could not cleanse the impurities (called sin) in our lives by ourselves. No amount of good deeds would accomplish this. We realized that only through accepting the sacrifice of Jesus Christ could our sins be forgiven. We both trusted Jesus Christ as our Savior in 1985 and we believe our names were forever written in the Lamb's Book of Life at that time.

Shortly thereafter, we joined Harrison Street Bible Church in Oak Park, Illinois. The church's senior pastor, John Blakemore, was originally from Olive Branch, a small town in southern Illinois. Pastor John felt compassion for that area even though he was working in Oak Park. Through Pastor John's contacts, a 40,000 square-foot dilapidated school building in Thebes, a town near Olive Branch, was donated to Harrison Street Bible Church in 1980. Harrison Street Bible Church hoped to use this building for ministry.

Pastor John's son, Peter, returned to Oak Park to co-pastor Harrison Street Bible Church after receiving theological training at Bob Jones University. Pastor Peter and his family soon became some of our closest friends and confidants. Pastor Peter was the kindest man my wife and I have known. At his encouragement, we started a charity Natural Medicine clinic at Harrison Street Bible Church in 1991. This clinic met in the church basement and was staffed by volunteers.

In early 1993, Marion and I decided we needed to get away. What could be farther away than Thebes, Illinois, which is a mere 400 miles away from Chicago and located in the middle of nowhere? We got much more than we bargained for by the end of the trip. We ended up buying a 120-acre farm. We named the property after Pastor John's favorite song: "Beulah Land." It comes from Isaiah 62:4: "No longer will they call you Deserted, or name your land Desolate. But you will be called Hephzibah, and your land Beulah; for the LORD will take delight in you, and your land will be married."

This verse describes the restoration of the relationship between God and His people Israel. We felt that this land would also be restored.

In late 1993, the first Beulah Land Natural Medicine Clinic was held in the basement of the First Baptist Church in Thebes, Illinois. Beulah Land Natural Medicine Clinic is staffed by volunteers from all over the United States. The doctors include Kurt Ehling, D.C., a chiropractic physician from Morton, Illinois; Rodney Van Pelt, M.D., an orthopedic medicine specialist from Ukiah, California; and myself. The clinic offers complete nutritional counseling, natural hormone treatments, chiropractic manipulation, physiotherapy, Metabolic Typing, intravenous therapies, and, of course, Prolotherapy.

The clinic is an outreach ministry to help people the way Jesus did. Most people sought help from Jesus for physical illnesses. This is well illustrated in the Bible verse Matthew 4:23: "Jesus went throughout Galilee, teaching in the synagogues, preaching the good news of the kingdom, and healing every disease and sickness among the people."[2] He never charged them. He often gave them encouragement to live justly and uprightly and to commit their ways to God. I believe Beulah Land Natural Medicine Clinic is doing just that.

It is my dream for Beulah Land Natural Medicine Clinic to become a renowned medical center like the Mayo Clinic, except Natural Medicine would be practiced and people could receive the best treatments **always free of charge**. Because of the devastating effects of chronic illnesses, many people do not have the resources to receive natural treatments. Beulah Land is a place where treatment is offered free of charge and hope is given. We continue to provide care in the church basement. We look forward to what God has in store for the future.

Beulah Land can always use additional assistance. If you would like to help as a volunteer, counselor, carpenter, electrician, nurse, or doctor please let us know. If you would like treatment, the clinic is available to you.

If someone out there is a millionaire and wants to donate money so we can buy land and start the clinic building, please stop reading and call me immediately at (708) 848-7789.

To contact Beulah Land Natural Medicine Clinic, write to Beulah Land, P.O. Box 197, Thebes, IL 62990, or contact my office in Oak Park, Illinois.

Letters of Appreciation

Because of the success of Prolotherapy in relieving pain, I have quite a collection of thank you letters from all over the country and around the world, from patients and doctors who have learned this technique. I enjoy receiving these letters. Believe it or not, seldom do physicians hear the words "thank you." These are words that we all need to say more often.

I would like to take this opportunity to say thank you to the patients that have had enough confidence in me to let me be their doctor and utilize the technique of Prolotherapy to relieve their pain. I would also like to say thank you to the physicians who had enough confidence in me to trust me to teach them this technique.

I hope you enjoy these thank you letters that have been an encouragement to me. I hope some day to receive a thank you letter from you when you Prolo your pain away.

Sincerely,

Ross A. Hauser M.D.

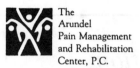

The
Arundel
Pain Management
and Rehabilitation
Center, P.C.

William Tham, M.D.
Susan Zimmerman, M.D.
Board Certified
Physical Medicine and Rehabilitation
Electromyography™
Medical Acupuncture
Pain Management
Spine Care

February 28, 1995

Ross Hauser, M.D.
715 Lake Street
Suite 600
Olde Parke, IL 60301

Dear Dr. Hauser:

I just wanted to drop you a note and let you know how successful we
have been with the prolotherapy treatments. Since learning the
technique from you at the prolotherapy seminar, we have treated
nearly 100 patients. We have been able to get excellent results on
patients that have had chronic pain for many years. I have one
patient that had multiple back surgeries, including fusion and
instrumentation, that has reported a good 90% improvement in her
pain complaints since receiving a course of two prolotherapy
treatments using your recommended solution of Dextrose mixed with
Lidocaine. What amazes me is that she continues to have
improvement on a long term basis. This treatment obviously is not
a quick fix approach. I cannot image the savings in terms of
health care dollars for these chronic pain patients with the use of
prolotherapy.

Sincerely,

William Tham, M.D.

WT/ky

706 Giddings Avenue, Suite 2B, Annapolis, MD 21401, (410) 268-2943
200 Hospital Drive, Suite 102, Glen Burnie, MD 21061, (410) 761-0030

February 19, 1997

RECEIVED MAR 1 0 1997

Dr. Ross Hauser
Caring Medical & Rehabilitation Service, S.C.
715 Lake Street, Suite 600
Oak Park, Illinois 60301
Tel (708) 848-7789   REF:DRRUSS.WPS

Dear Dr. Ross Hauser:

First I would like to say may God bless you and your wife for the wonderful work that you do for the Lord!
I would like to give my personal testimony of how God used you, and the medicine that you gave me to cure me of back pain.

I had low back pain for more than eight years. Through I visited many doctors here in Mexico, no one had a definitive cure for my problem. Throughout this time I took several medicine- they were just to control the pain. They did not help the problem.

I am really grateful that a brother in Christ that work for the Institute of Basic Principles gave me your name, address and phone number so I could visit you in Chicago. My diagnosis is Lumbar Scoliosis. Last August 1996 in Chicago I received my first prolotherapy treatment of forthy injections. My second treatment was in Mexico City December 1996, I received twenty injections there. Now I do not have any pain at all. Finally I can rest at night and have a normal life without pain. In January 1997, Dr. Gerardo Cajero also injected my kness for pain that I was having in them.

The Lord has blessed us a lot here in Mexico. Dr. Cajero has many patients in Mexico City and in Monterrey. The mexican people are really grateful to you because you invest your time in training Dr. Cajero.

Also we are really interested in any information that you might have on conferences or medical literature to support this treatment, which we can present to the Mexican Medical Asociation. Dr. Cajero is very interested in forming a Society of Prolotherapy here in Mexico. Please pray about that.

Again, thank you so much for your help and for willingness to serve the Lord and others.

With Love,

Miriam Morales
Miriam Morales

June 16, 1997

Dear Dr. Hauser,

First I would like to thank you for bringing your Clinic to Southern Illinois.

I was diagnosed with Osteoarthritis in both knees and lower back last year. I was in severe pain and almost to the point of not being able to walk or do simple household tasks. The Specialist had told me I would have to have my right knee replaced or I would probably not be able to walk without severe pain. So I was almost willing to try anything. I went to the Beulah Land Clinic in Thebes at the suggestion of a friend and am very glad I did. I had Prolotherapy on Both knees and lower back. I have had three treatments so far and am virtually pain free in my left knee and lower back. I still have some pain in my right knee, but not even a quarter of what it used to be. I am back to walking any where from three to five miles a day, so feel very fortunate. I would highly recommend this treatment to any one who has a problem like mine.

Again Thank-You very much and am looking forward to your return Trip to Southern Illinois

Yours Truly,
Sharon Calvert

August 15, 1997

Rita S. Mueller

Dear Dr. Hauser,

After a dozen e-rays and a MRI Scan, the doctors said the pain in my hip was probably do to a fall from the year before and hereditary arthritis that had settled in my joints. The pain became so great that I had to stop all physical activity and for weeks at a time I could barely walk. Placing any weight on the leg would cause tears to come to my eyes. After a year and a half of anti-inflammatory medication and pain pills, the doctors told me my only option was a hip replacement. A new hip would last between 15 and 20 years and cost between 16 to 20 thousand dollars. At age 41 that was not what I wanted to hear. My physical therapist gave me your name and would tell me nothing else but that you had a treatment that might help me.

I talked to you for an hour about prolotherapy and how prolotherapy along with vitamins, proper nutrition, and exercise would help my body heal itself. I felt I had nothing to lose, so I had the treatment that day. One week later I was riding my bike ten miles a day and my husband and I started ballroom dancing again. My husband was in shock because only the week before he had to help me get up the stairs. As I resumed all my normal activities, I felt those other doctors had stolen a year of my life from me. I had only one prolotherapy treatment.

It now has been three years since I had prolotherapy. We took a three week hiking trip to Alaska. We hiked a mountain to the top of a glacier field and as I stood there, which to me was the top of the world, I laughed at those doctors who said hip replacement and I thanked God for having met you and prolotherapy.

I wanted to thank you again and only wish more people could be made aware of alternatives to surgery. I just got lucky that my physical therapist new and believed in your work.

Sincerely,

Rita S. Mueller

NOTES

ACKNOWLEDGEMENTS
[1] The Holy Bible, New International Version, Psalm 71:14-16.

DEDICATION
[1] The Holy Bible, New International Version, Matthew 11:4-5.
[2] The Holy Bible, New International Version, Matthew 25:34-40.

CHAPTER 2
Introduction: The Technique and Its History
[1] Schneider, R. "Fatality after injection of sclerosing agent to precipitate fibro-osseous pro-liferation." *Journal of the American Medical Association.* 1959; 170:1768-1772.
[2] An abstract of a poster presentation (poster #49) at the 59th Annual Assembly of the American Academy of Physical Medicine and Rehabilitation printed in the *Archives of Physical Medicine and Rehabilitation.*
[3] Kim, M. "Myofascial trigger point therapy: comparison of dextrose, water, saline, and lidocaine." *Archives of Physical Medicine and Rehabilitation.* 1997; 78:1028.
[4] Klein, R. "A randomized double-blind trial of dextrose-glycerine-phenol injections for chronic, low back pain." *Journal of Spinal Disorders.* 1993; 6:23-33.
[5] Ongley, M. "A new approach to the treatment of chronic low back pain." *Lancet.* 1987; 2:143-146.
[6] Travell, J. *Myofascial Pain and Dysfunction.* Baltimore, MD: Williams and Wilkins, 1983, pp. 103-164.
[7] Wiesel, S. "A study of computer-related assisted tomography 1. The incidence of positive CAT scans in an asymptomatic group of patients." *Spine.* 1984; 9:549-551.
[8] From a phone conversation with C. Everett Koop, M.D., on May 16, 1987.
[9] Boyd, Nathaniel. *Stay Out of the Hospital.* New York, NY: The Two Continents Publishing Group, Ltd., 1976, pp. 125-128.
[10] Ibid.

CHAPTER 3
Why Prolotherapy Works
[1] Hackett, G. *Ligament and Tendon Relaxation Treated by Prolotherapy.* Third Edition. Springfield, IL: Charles C. Thomas Publisher, 1958, p. 5.

[2]   Babcock, P. et al. *Webster's Third New International Dictionary.* Springfield, MA: G.& C. Merriam Co., 1971, p. 1815.

[3]   Browner, B. *Skeletal Trauma. Volume 1.* Philadelphia, PA: W.B. Saunders Company, 1992, pp. 87-88.

[4]   Deese, J. "Compressive neuropathies of the lower extremity." *The Journal of Musculoskeletal Medicine.* 1988; November: 68-91.

[5]   Kayfetz, D. "Occipital-cervical (whiplash) injuries treated by prolotherapy." *Medical Trail Technique Quarterly.* 1963; June: 9-29

[6]   Rhalmi, S. "Immunohistochemical study of nerves in lumbar spine ligaments." *Spine.* 1993; 18:264-267.

[7]   Ahmed, M. "Neuropeptide Y, tyrosine hydroxylase and vasoactive intestinal polypeptide immunoreactive nerve fibers in the vertebral bodies, discs, dura mater, and spinal ligaments of the rat lumbar spine." *Spine.* 1993; 18:268-273.

[8]   Hackett G., Hemwall, G., and Montgomery, G. *Ligament and Tendon Relaxation Treated by Prolotherapy.* Fifth Edition. Oak Park, IL: Gustav A. Hemwall, Publisher, 1993, p. 20.

[9]   Rhalmi, S. "Immunohistochemical study of nerves in lumbar spine ligaments." *Spine.* 1993; 18:264-267.

[10]   Ahmed, M. "Neuropeptide Y, tyrosine hydroxylase and vasoactive intestinal polypeptide-immunoreactive nerve fibers in the vertebral bodies, discs, dura mater, and spinal ligaments of the rat lumbar spine." *Spine.* 1993; 18:268-273.

[11]   Robbins, S. *Pathologic Basis of Disease.* Third Edition. Philadelphia, PA: W.B. Saunders Co., 1984, p. 40.

CHAPTER 4
Prolotherapy Provides Results

[1]   Hackett, G. *Ligament and Tendon Relaxation Treated by Prolotherapy.* Third Edition. Springfield, IL: Charles C. Thomas Publisher, 1958, p. 5 and Hackett, G. "Low back pain." *The British Journal of Physical Medicine.* 1956; 19:25-33.

[2]   Hackett, G. "Referred pain and sciatica in diagnosis of low back disability" *Journal of the American Medical Association.* 1957; 163:183-185.

[3]   Hackett, G. "Joint stabilization." *American Journal of Surgery.* 1955; 89:968-973.

[4]   Hackett, G. "Referred pain from low back ligament disability." AMA Archives of Surgery. 73:878-883, November 1956.

[5]   Liu, Y. "An in situ study of the influence of a sclerosing solution in rabbit medial collateral ligaments and its junction strength." *Connective Tissue Research.* 1983; 2:95-102.

[6]   Maynard, J. "Morphological and biomechanical effects of sodium morrhuate on tendons." *Journal of Orthopaedic Research.* 1985; 3:236-248.

[7]   Ibid.

[8]   Klein, R. "Proliferant injections for low back pain: histologic changes of injected ligaments and objective measures of lumbar spine mobility before and after treatment." *Journal of Neurology, Orthopedic Medicine and Surgery.* 1989; 10:141-144.

[9]   "Interview with Thomas Dorman, M.D." *Nutrition & Healing.* 1994; pp. 5-6.

[10]   Dorman, T. "Treatment for spinal pain arising in ligaments using prolotherapy: A retrospective study." *Journal of Orthopaedic Medicine.* 1991; 13(1):13-19.

[11] Ongley, M. and Dorman T. et al. "Ligament instability of knees: A new approach to treatment." *Manual Medicine.* 1988; 3:152-154.

[12] Klein R. "A randomized double-blind trial of dextrose-glycerine-phenol injections for chronic, low back pain." *Journal of Spinal Disorders.* 1993; 6:23-33.

[13] Ongley, M. "A new approach to the treatment of chronic low back pain." *Lancet.* 1987; 2:143-146.

[14] Schwartz, R. "Prolotherapy: A literature review and retrospective study." *Journal of Neurology, Orthopedic Medicine, and Surgery.* 1991;12:220-223.

[15] Wilkinson, H. "Broad Spectrum Approach to the Failed Back." Lecture presentation at the American College of Osteopathic Pain Management and Sclerotherapy meeting on May 3, 1997.

CHAPTER 5
Answers to Common Questions About Prolotherapy

[1] Meyers, A. "Prolotherapy treatment of low back pain and sciatica." *Bulletin of the Hospital for Joint Disease.* 1961; 22:1.

[2] Woo, S. "Injury and repair of the musculoskeletal soft tissues. *American Academy of Orthopedic Surgeons.* 1987.

[3] Mankin, H. "Localization of tritiated thymidine in articular cartilage of rabbits inhibits growth in immature cartilage." *Journal of Bone & Joint Surgery.* 1962; 44A:682.

[4] Butler, D. "Biomechanics of ligaments and tendons." *Exercise and Sports Scientific Review.* 1975; 6:125.

[5] Bland, J. *Disorders of the Cervical Spine.* Philadelphia, PA: W.B. Saunders, 1987.

[6] Letter written April 20, 1976 by Carell Hutchingson, Jr., M.D., as chairman of the Subcommittee on Insurance Mediation for the Chicago Medical Society, CMS No. 76-M-005.

[7] Letter written November 1, 1979 by Michael Treister, M.D., as chairman of the Medical Practice Committee for the Chicago Medical Society regarding CMS File 79-G-069.

[8] Letter written November 5, 1987 by Peter C. Pulos, M.D., as chairman of the Medical Practice Committee for the Chicago Medical Society regarding Claim No. 725514.

[9] Reeves, K. "Technique of Prolotherapy." From *Physiatric Procedures in Clinical Practice.* Philadelphia, PA: Hanley and Belfus, Inc., 1994, pp. 57-70.

[10] Reeves, K. "Prolotherapy, present and future applications in soft-tissue pain and disability." *Physical Medicine and Rehabilitation Clinics of North America.* 1995; 6:917-925.

[11] Dorman, T. *Diagnosis and Injection Techniques in Orthopedic Medicine.* Baltimore, MD: Williams and Wilkins, 1991.

[12] Faber, W., and Walker, M. *Instant Pain Relief.* Milwaukee, WI: Biological Publications, 1991.

[13] Faber, W., and Walker, M. *Pain, Pain Go Away.* San Jose, CA: ISHI Press International, 1990.

[14] Butler, D. "Biomechanics of ligaments and tendons." *Exercise & Sports Scientific Review.* 1975; 6:125.

[15] Tipton, C. "Influence of immobilization, training, exogenous hormones, and surgical repair of knee ligaments from hypophysectomized rats. *American Journal of Physiology.* 1971; 221:1114.

[16] Nachemson, A. "Some mechanical properties of the third human lumbar interlaminar lig-

ament." *Journal of Biomechanics*. 1968; 1:211.

[17] Akeson, W. "The Connective Tissue Response to Immobility: An Accelerated Aging Response." *Experimental Gerontology*. 1968; 3:239.

[18] Travell, J. *Myofascial Pain and Dysfunction*. Baltimore, MD: Williams and Wilkins, 1983, pp. 103-164.

[19] Schumacher, H. *Primer on the Rheumatic Diseases*. Tenth Edition. Atlanta, GA: Arthritis Foundation, 1993, pp. 8-11.

[20] Ballard, W. "Biochemical aspects of aging and degeneration in the invertebral disc." *Contemporary Orthopaedics*. 1992; 24:453-458.

[21] Jacobs, R. *Pathogenesis of Idiopathic Scoliosis*. Chicago, IL: Scoliosis Research Society, 1984, pp. 107-118.

[22] Crowninsheild, R. "The strength and failure characteristics of rat medial collateral ligaments." Journal of Trauma. 1976; 16:99.

[23] Travell, J. *Myofascial Pain and Dysfunction*. Baltimore, MD: Williams and Wilkins, 1983, pp. 103-164.

[24] Tipton, C. "Response of adrenalectomized rats to exercise." *Endocrinology*. 1972; 91:573.

[25] Tipton, C. "Response of thyroidectomized rats to training." *American Journal of Physiology*. 1972; 215:1137.

[26] Bucci, L. *Nutrition Applied to Injury Rehabilitation and Sports Medicine*. Boca Raton, FL: CRC Press, 1995, pp. 167-176.

[27] Batmanghelidj, F. *Your Body's Many Cries for Water*. Second Edition. Falls Church, VA: Global Health Solutions, Inc., 1996, pp. 8-11.

[28] Welbourne, T. "Increased plasma bicarbonate and growth hormone after an oral glutamine load." *American Journal of Clinical Nutrition*. 1995; pp. 1058-1061.

[29] Hurson, M. "Metabolic effects of arginine in a healthy elderly population." *Journal of Parenteral and Enteral Nutrition*. 1995; pp. 227-230.

[30] Dominguez, R. and Gajda, R. *Total Body Training*. East Dundee, IL: Moving Force Systems, 1982, pp. 33-37.

[31] Laros, G. "Influence of physical activity on ligament insertions in the knees of dogs." *Journal of Bone and Joint Surgery* (Am). 1971; 53:275.

[32] Hunter, L. *Rehabilitation of the Injured Knee*. St. Louis, MO: The C.V. Mosby Company, 1984.

[33] Arnoczky, S. "Meniscal degeneration due to knee instability: an experimental study in the dog." *Trans. Orthop. Res. Soc.* 1979; 4:79.

[34] Hunter, L. *Rehabilitation of the Injured Knee*. St. Louis, MO: The C.V. Mosby Company, 1984.

[35] Arnoczky, S. "Meniscal degeneration due to knee instability: an experimental study in the dog." *Trans. Orthop. Res. Soc.* 1979; 4:79.

[36] Tipton, C. "The influence of physical activity on ligaments and tendons." *Med. Sci. Sports*. 1975; 7:165.

[37] Woo, S. "Effect of immobilization and exercise on strength characteristics of bone-medial collateral ligament-bone complex." *Am. Soc. Mech. Eng. Symp.* 1979; 32:62.

[38] Hunter, L. *Rehabilitation of the Injured Knee*. St. Louis, MO: The C.V. Mosby Company, 1984.

[39] Noyes, F. "Biomechanics of anterior cruciate ligament failure: an analysis of strain rate sensitivity and mechanism of failure in primates." *Journal of Bone & Joint Surgery*. 1974; 56A:236.

[40] Noyes, F. "Biomechanics of ligament failure: an analysis of immobilization, exercise and reconditioning effects in primates." *Journal of Bone & Joint Surgery*. 1974; 56A:1406.

[41] Laros, G. "Influence of physical activity on ligament insertions in the knees of dogs." *Journal of Bone & Joint Surgery* (Am). 1971; 53A:275.

[42] Hunter, L. *Rehabilitation of the Injured Knee.* St. Louis, MO: The C.V. Mosby Company, 1984.

[43] Akeson, W. "Immobility effects on synovial joints: The pathomechanics of joint contracture." *Biorheology.* 1980; 17:95.

[44] Ho, S. "Comparison of various icing times in decreasing bone metabolism and blood flow in the knee." *The American Journal of Sports Medicine.* 1990; 18:376-378.

[45] McGaw, W. "The effect of tension on collagen remodeling by fibroblasts: a sterological ultrastructural study." *Connective Tissue Research.* 1986; 14:229-235.

[46] Bucci, L. *Nutrition Applied to Injury Rehabilitation and Sports Medicine.* Boca Raton, FL: CRC Press, 1995, pp. 167-176.

[47] Hardy, M. "The biology of scar formation." *Physical Therapy.* 1989; 69:12.

[48] Mishra, D. "Anti-inflammatory medication after muscle injury: A treatment resulting in short-term improvement but subsequent loss of muscle function." *Journal of Bone & Joint Surgery.* 1995; 77A:1510-1519.

[49] Brandt, K. "Should osteoarthritis be treated with nonsteroidal anti-inflammatory drugs?" *Rheumatic Disease Clinics of North America.* 1993; 19:697-712.

[50] Brandt, K. "The effects of salicylates and other nonsteoridal anti-inflammatory drugs on articular cartilage." *American Journal of Medicine.* 1984; 77:65-69.

[51] Obeid, G. "Effect of ibuprofen on the healing and remodeling of bone and articular cartilage in the rabbit temporomandibular joint." *Journal of Oral and Maxillofacial Surgeons.* 1992; pp. 843-850.

[52] Dupont, M. "The efficacy of anti-inflammatory medication in the treatment of the acutely sprained ankle." *The American Journal of Sports Medicine.* 1987; 15:41-45.

[53] Newman, N. "Acetabular bone destruction related to nonsteroidal anti-inflammatory drugs." *The Lancet.* 1985; July 6:11-13.

[54] Serup, J. and Oveson, J. "Salicylate arthropathy: accelerated coxarthrosis during long-term treatment with acetyl salicylic acid." *Praxis.* 1981; 70:359.

[55] Ronningen, H. and Langeland, N. "Indomethacin treatment in osteoarthritis of the hip joint." *Acta Orthopedica Scandanavia.* 1979; 50:169-174.

[56] Newman, N. "Acetabular bone destruction related to nonsteroidal anti-inflammatory drugs." *The Lancet.* 1985; July 6:11-13.

[57] Serup, J. and Ovesen, J. "Salicylate arthropathy: accelerated coxarthrosis during long-term treatment with acetyl salicylic acid." *Praxis.* 1981; 70:359.

[58] Ronningen, H. and Langeland, N. "Indomethacin treatment in osteoarthritis of the hip joint. *Acta Orthopedica Scandanavia.* 1979; 50:169-174.

[59] Akil, M., Amos, R.S., and Stewart, P. "Infertility may sometimes be associated with NSAID consumption." *British Journal of Rheumatism.* 1996; 35:76-78.

[60] Wrenn, R. "An experimental study of the effect of cortisone on the healing process and

tensile strength of tendons." *The Journal of Bone and Joint Surgery.* 1954; 36A:588-601.

[61]   Truhan, A. "Corticosteroids: A review with emphasis on complications of prolonged systemic therapy." *Annals of Allergy.* 1989; 62:375-390.

[62]   Roenigk, R. *Dermatologic Surgery.* Marcel Dekker, Inc., p. 155.

[63]   Davis, G. "Adverse effects of corticosteroids: 11." *Systemic Clinical Dermatology.* 1986; 4(1):161-169.

[64]   Gogia, P. "Hydrocortisone and exercise effects on articular cartilage in rats." *Archives of Physical Medicine and Rehabilitation.* 1993; 74:463-467.

[65]   Chandler, G.N. "Deleterious effect of intra-articular hydrocortisone." *Lancet.* 1958; 2:661-63.

[66]   Wiley, R. *Biobalance.* Tacoma, WA: Life Sciences Press, 1989, pp. 7-18.

[67]   Reams, C. *Choose Life or Death.* Fifth Edition. Tampa, FL: Holistic Laboratories, 1990, pp. 80-85.

[68]   Wiley, R. *Biobalance.* Tacoma, WA: Life Sciences Press, 1989, pp. 7-18.

[69]   Sears, B. *The Zone.* New York, NY: HarperCollins Publishers, Inc., 1995.

CHAPTER 6
Prolotherapy, Inflammation, and Healing: What's the Connection?

[1]   Robbins, S. *Pathologic Basis of Disease.* Third Edition. Philadelphia, PA: W.B. Saunders Co., 1984, p. 40.

[2]   Greenfield, B. *Rehabilitation of the Knee: A Problem Solving Approach.* F.A. Davis Co., 1993.

[3]   Woo, S. "Injury and repair of the musculoskeletal soft tissues." *American Academy of Orthopedic Surgeons.* 1987.

[4]   Mankin, H. "Localization of tritiated thymidine in articular cartilage of rabbits inhibits growth in immature cartilage." *Journal of Bone & Joint Surgery.* 1962; 44A:682.

[5]   Robbins, S. *Pathologic Basis of Disease.* Third Edition. Philadelphia, PA: W.B. Saunders Co., 1984, p. 40.

[6]   Greenfield, B. *Rehabilitation of the Knee: A Problem Solving Approach.* F.A. Davis Co., 1993.

[7]   Woo, S. "Injury and repair of the musculoskeletal soft tissues." *American Academy of Orthopedic Surgeons.* 1987.

[8]   Benedetti, R. "Clinical results of simultaneous adjacent interdigital neurectomy in the foot." *Foot Ankle International.* 1996; 17:264-268.

CHAPTER 7
Prolo Your Back Pain Away

[1]   Boden, S. "Abnormal magnetic-resonance scans of the lumbar spine in asymptomatic subjects." *The Journal of Bone and Joint Surgery.* 1990; 72A:403-408.

[2]   Jensen, M. "Magnetic resonance imaging of the lumbar spine in people without back pain." *The New England Journal of Medicine.* 1994; 331:69-73.

[3]   Boden, S. "Abnormal magnetic-resonance scans of the lumbar spine in asymptomatic subjects." *The Journal of Bone and Joint Surgery.* 1990; 72A:403-408.

[4]   Jensen, M. "Magnetic resonance imaging of the lumbar spine in people without back

pain." *The New England Journal of Medicine.* 1994; 331:69-73.

[5] Hackett, G. "Shearing injury to the sacroiliac joint." *The Journal of the International College of Surgeons.* 1954; 22:631-639.

[6] Bellamy, N. "What do we know about the sacroiliac joint?" *Seminars in Arthritis and Rheumatism.* 1983; 12:282-313.

[7] Paris, S. "Physical signs of instability." *Spine.* 1985; 10:277-279.

[8] Hackett, G. "Shearing injury to the sacroiliac joint." *The Journal of the International College of Surgeons.* 1954; 22:631-639.

[9] Mueller, R. *"Anesthesia" in Current Surgical Diagnosis and Treatment.* Seventh Edition. Los Altes, CA. 1983, pp. 162-169.

[10] Burton, C. "Conservative management of low back pain." *Postgraduate Medicine.* 5:168-183.

[11] Merriman, J. "Prolotherapy versus operative fusion in the treatment of joint instability of the spine and pelvis." *Journal of the International College of Surgeons.* 1964; 42:150-159.

[12] Ibid.

[13] Maynard, J. "Morphological and biomechanical effects of sodium morrhuate on tendons." *Journal of Orthopaedic Research.* 1985; 3:236-248.

[14] Turner, J. et al. "Patient outcomes after lumbar spinal fusions." *Journal of the American Medical Association.* 1992; 286:907-910.

[15] Schwarzer, A. "The sacroiliac joint in chronic low back pain." *Spine.* 1995; 20:31-37.

[16] Adams, R. and Victor, M., ed. *Principles of Neurology.* Fourth Edition. St. Louis, MO: McGraw Hill, 1989, pp. 737-738.

[17] Hoffman, G. "Spinal arachnoiditis – what is the clinical spectrum?" *Spine.* 1983; 8:538-540.

[18] Guyer, D. "The long-range prognosis of arachnoiditis." *Spine.* 1989; 14:1332-1341.

[19] Jackson, A. "Does degenerative disease of the lumbar spine cause arachnoiditis? A magnetic resonance study and review of the literature. *The British Journal of Radiology.* 1994; 64:840-847.

[20] Guyer, D. "The long-range prognosis of arachnoiditis." *Spine.* 1989; 14:1332-1341.

[21] U.S. Preventive Services Task Force. "Screening for adolescent idiopathic scoliosis." *Journal of the American Medical Association.* 1993; 269:2667-2672.

[22] Bradford, D. "Adult scoliosis." *Clinical Orthopaedics and Related Research.* 1988; 229:70-86.

[23] Gunnoe, B. "Adult idiopathic scoliosis." *Orthopaedic Review.* 1990; 19:35-43.

[24] Keim, H. "Adult scoliosis and its management." *Orthopaedic Review.* 1981; 10:41-48.

[25] Winter, R. "Pain patterns in adult scoliosis." *Orthopedic Clinics of North America.* 1988; 19:339-345.

CHAPTER 8
Prolo Your Headache, Neck, TMJ, Ear, and Mouth Pain Away

[1] Bellamy, N. "What do we know about the sacroiliac joint?" *Seminars in Arthritis and Rheumatism.* 1983; 12:282-313.

[2] Barré, J. *Rev. Neurol.* 1926; 33:1246.

[3] Tamura, T. "Cranial symptoms after cervical injury–aetiology and treatment of the Barré-Lieou Syndrome." *The Journal of Bone and Joint Surgery*, 1989; 71B:283-287.

⁴   Bland, J. *Disorders of the Cervical Spine*. Philadelphia, PA: W.B. Saunders, 1987.

⁵   Kayfetz, D. "Whiplash injury and other ligamentous headache–its management with pro-lotherapy." *Headache*. 1963; 3:1-8.

⁶   Claussen, C.F. and Claussen E. "Neurootological contributions to the diagnostic follow-up after whiplash injuries." *Acta Otolaryngology (Stockh)*. 1995; Suppl 520:53-56.

⁷   Hackett, G. "Prolotherapy for headache." *Headache*. 1962; 1:3-11.

⁸   Hackett, G. "Prolotherapy in whiplash and low back pain." *Postgraduate Medicine*. 1960; pp. 214-219.

⁹   Kayfetz, D. "Whiplash injury and other ligamentous headache–its management with pro-lotherapy." *Headache*. 1963; 3:1-8.

¹⁰   Merriman, J. Presentation at the Hackett Foundation Prolotherapy Meeting, Indianapolis, Indiana, October 1995.

¹¹   Caviness, V. "Current concepts in headache." *The New England Journal of Medicine*. 1980; 302:446-450.

¹²   Darnell, M. "A proposed chronology of events for forward head posture." *The Journal of Craniomandibular Practice*. 1983; 1:49-54.

¹³   Rocabado, M. "Biomechanical relationship of the cranial, cervical and hyoid regions." *Physical Therapy*. 1983; 1:62-66.

¹⁴   Schultz, L. "A treatment for subluxation of the temporomandibular joint." *Journal of the American Medical Association*. September 25, 1937; pp. 1032-1035.

¹⁵   Schultz, L. "Twenty years experience in treating hypermobility of the temporomandibular joints." *The American Journal of Surgery*. 1956; 92:925-928.

¹⁶   Cheshire, W. "Botulinum toxin in the treatment of myofascial pain syndrome." *Pain*. 1994; 59:65-69.

¹⁷   *Headache Relief Newsletter*, Edition 13, Philadelphia, PA: The Pain Center, 1995.

¹⁸   Thigpen, C. "The styloid process." *Trans American Laryngological Rhinology Otology Association*. 1932; 28:408-412.

¹⁹   Eagle, W. "Elongated styloid process." *Archives of Otolaryngology*. 1937; 25:584-587.

²⁰   Shankland, W. "Differential diagnosis of headaches." *Journal of Craniomandibular Practice*. 1986; 4:47-53.

²¹   Ernest, E. "Three disorders that frequently cause temporomandibular joint pain: internal derangement, temporal tendonitis, and Ernest syndrome. *Journal of Neurological Orthopedic Surgery*. 1986; 7:189-191.

²²   Shankland, W. "Ernest syndrome as a consequence of stylomandibular ligament injury: A report of 68 patients." *The Journal of Prosthetic Dentistry*. 1987; 57:501-506.

²³   Wong, E. "Temporal headaches and associated symptoms relating to the styloid process and its attachments. *Annals of Academic Medicine Singapore*. 1995; 24:124-128.

CHAPTER 9
Prolo Your Shoulder Pain Away

¹   Matsen, F. "Anterior glenohumeral instability." *Clinics in Sports Medicine*. 1983; 2:319-336.

²   Bonafede, R. "Shoulder pain." *Postgraduate Medicine*. 1987; 82:185-193.

³   Frieman, B. "Rotator cuff disease: A review of diagnosis, pathophysiology, and current trends in treatment." *Archives of Physical Medicine and Rehabilitation*. 1994; 75:604-609.

[4] Ibid.

[5] Andersen, L. "Shoulder pain in hemiplegia." *The American Journal of Occupational Therapy*. 1985; 39:11-18.

[6] Scott, J. "Injuries to the acromioclavicular joint." *Injury: The British Journal of Accident Surgery*. 1967; 5:13-18.

[7] Butters, K. "Office evaluation and management of the shoulder impingement syndrome." *Orthopedic Clinics of North America*. 1988; 19:755-765.

[8] Chandnani, V. "MRI findings in asymptomatic shoulders: A blind analysis using symptomatic shoulders as controls." *Clinical Imaging*. 1992; 16:25-30.

[9] Neumann, C. "MR imaging of the shoulder: appearance of the supraspinatus tendon in asymptomatic volunteers." *American Journal of Radiology*. 1992; 158:1281-1287.

[10] Sher, J. "Abnormal findings on magnetic resonance images of asymptomatic shoulders." *The Journal of Bone and Joint Surgery*. 1995; 77A:10-15.

[11] Neumann, C. "MR imaging of the shoulder: appearance of the supraspinatus tendon in asymptomatic volunteers." *American Journal of Radiology*. 1992; 158:1281-1287.

[12] Ibid.

[13] Sher, J. "Abnormal findings on magnetic resonance images of asymptomatic shoulders." *The Journal of Bone & Joint Surgery*. 1995; 77A:10-15.

CHAPTER 10
Prolo Your Elbow, Wrist, and Hand Pain Away

[1] Armstrong, T. "Upper-extremity pain in the workplace – Role of usage in causality in clinical concepts." from *Regional Musculoskeletal Illness*. Grune and Straton, Inc., 1987, pp. 333-354.

[2] Dominguez, R. and Gajda, R. *Total Body Training*. East Dundee, IL: Moving Force Systems, 1982, pp. 33-37.

[3] Bucci, L. *Nutrition Applied to Injury Rehabilitation and Sports Medicine*. Boca Raton, FL: CRC Press, 1995, pp. 167-176.

[4] Cooney, W. "Anatomy and mechanics of carpal instability." *Surgical Rounds for Orthopedics*. 1989; pp. 5-24.

[5] Ibid.

[6] Kozin, S. "Injuries to the perilunar carpus." *Orthopaedic Review*. 1992; 21:435-448.

[7] Waters, P. "Unusual arthritic disorders in the hand: part 1." *Surgical Rounds for Orthopaedics*. 1990; pp. 15-20.

[8] Laseter, G. "Management of the stiff hand: A practical approach." *Orthopedic Clinics of North America*. 1983; 14:749-765.

CHAPTER 11
Prolo Your Groin, Hip, and Knee Pain Away

[1] Meisenbach, R. "Sacro-iliac relaxation; with analysis of eighty-four cases." *Surgery, Gynecology and Obstetrics*. 1911; 12:411-434.

[2] Ibid.

[3] Hirschberg, G. "Iliolumbar syndrome as a common cause of low back pain: diagnosis and prognosis." *Archives of Physical Medicine and Rehabilitation*. 1979; 60:415-419.

[4]   Schwarzer, A. "The sacroiliac joint in chronic low back pain. *Spine.* 1995; 20:31-37.

[5]   Friberg, O. "Clinical symptoms and biomechanics of lumbar spine and hip joint in leg length inequality." *Spine.* 1983; 18:643-651.

[6]   Cummings, G. "The effect of imposed leg length difference on pelvic bone symmetry. *Spine.* 1993; 18:368-373.

[7]   Ober, F. "The role of the iliotibial band and fascia lata as a factor in the causation of low-back disabilities and sciatica. *The Journal of Bone and Joint Surgery.* 1936; 18.

[8]   Swezey, R. "Pseudo-radiculopathy in subacute trochanteric bursitis of the subgluteus maximus bursa." *Archives of Physical Medicine and Rehabilitation.* 1976; 57:387-390.

[9]   Ober, F. "The role of the iliotibial band and fascia lata as a factor in the causation of low-back disabilities and sciatica. *The Journal of Bone and Joint Surgery.* 1936; 18.

[10] Schwartz, R. "Prolotherapy: a literature review and retrospective study." *Journal of Orthopaedic Medicine and Surgery.* 1991; 12:220-223.

[11] Peterson, L. *Sports Injuries, Their Prevention and Treatment.* Chicago, IL: Year Book Medical, 1986, pp. 18-63.

[12] Ongley, M. "Ligament instability of knees: A new approach to treatment." *Manual Medicine.* 1988; 3:152-154.

[13] Graham, G. "Early osteoarthritis in young sportsmen with severe anterolateral instability of the knee." *Injury: The British Journal of Accident Surgery.* 1988; 19:247-248.

[14] Ongley, M. "Ligament instability of knees: A new approach to treatment." *Manual Medicine.* 1988; 3:152-154.

[15] Hryhorowych, A. "Pes anserinus tendonitis: A major component of knee pain in elderly individuals with degenerative joint disease." Abstract at the American Academy of Physical Medicine and Rehabilitation meeting, November, 1993.

[16] Kidd, R. "Recent developments in the understanding of Osgood-Schlatter disease: A literature review." *The Journal of Orthopaedic Medicine.* 1993; 15:59-63.

CHAPTER 12
Prolo Your Ankle and Foot Pain Away

[1]   Mann, R. "Pain in the foot." *Postgraduate Medicine.* 1987; 82:154-174.

[2]   Mankin, H. "Localization of tritiated thymidine in articular cartilage of rabbits inhibits growth in immature cartilage." *Journal of Bone & Joint Surgery.* 1962; 44A:682.

[3]   Karr, S. "Subcalcaneal heel pain." *Orthopedic Clinics of North America.* 1994; 25:161-175.

[4]   Merriman, J. "Presentation at the Hackett Foundation Prolotherapy Meeting, Indianapolis, Indiana. October 1995.

[5]   Trevino, S. "Management of acute and chronic lateral ligament injuries of the ankle." Orthopedic Clinics of North America. 1994; 25:1-16.

[6]   Kirvela, O. "Treatment of painful neuromas with neurolytic blockade." *Pain.* 1990; 41:161-165.

[7]   Benedetti, R. "Clinical results of simultaneous adjacent interdigital neurectomy in the foot." *Foot Ankle International.* 1996; 17:264-268.

[8]   Deese, J. "Compressive neuropathies of the lower extremity." *The Journal of Musculoskeletal Medicine.* 1988; November:68-91

[9]   Hollinshead, W. *Functional Anatomy of the Limb and Back.* Fifth Edition. Philadelphia,

PA: W.B. Saunders, Co., pp. 316-338.

CHAPTER 13
Prolo Your Fibromyalgia Pain Away
[1] Yunnus, M. "Primary fibromyalgia syndrome and myofascial pain syndrome: Clinical features and muscle pathology." *Archives of Physical Medicine and Rehabilitation.* 1988; 69:451-454.
[2] Pillemer, S. *The Fibromyalgia Syndrome.* The Harworth Medical Press, Inc., 1994.
[3] Bennett, R. "Fibrositis" from *The Textbook of Rheumatology*, Third Edition, Philadelphia, PA: W.B. Saunders Co., 1987, pp. 541-553.
[4] Moldofsky, H. "Induction of neurasthenic musculoskeletal pain syndrome by selective sleep stage deprivation." *Psychosomatic Medicine.* 1976; 38:35.
[5] Buchwald, D. "Comparison of patients with chronic fatigue syndrome, fibromyalgia, and multiple chemical sensitivities." *Archives of Internal Medicine.* 1994; 154:2049-2053.
[6] Crofford, L. "Hypothalamic-pituitary-adrenal axis perturbations in patients with fibromyalgia." *Arthritis and Rheumatism.* 1994; 37:1583-1592.
[7] Goldenberg, D. "Do infections trigger fibromyalgia?" *Arthritis and Rheumatism.* 1993; 36:1489-1492.
[8] Travell, J. *Myofascial Pain and Dysfunction.* Baltimore, MD: Williams and Wilkins, 1983, pp. 103-164.
[9] Reeves, K. "Treatment of consecutive severe fibromyalgia patients with prolotherapy." *The Journal of Orthopaedic Medicine.* 1994; 16:84-89.
[10] McCarty, D. *Arthritis and Allied Conditions.* Twelfth Edition. Lea and Febiger, 1993.
[11] Kowitz, R. *Osteoarthritis.* Second Edition. Philadelphia, PA: W.B. Saunders, 1992.
[12] Travell, J. *Myofascial Pain and Dysfunction*, Baltimore, MD: Williams and Wilkins, 1983, pp. 103-164.
[13] Hong, C. "Difference in pain relief after trigger point injections in myofascial pain patients with and without fibromyalgia." *Archives of Physical Medicine and Rehabilitation.* 1996; 77:1161-1166.

CHAPTER 14
Prolo Your Arthritis Pain Away
[1] Christie, R. "The medical uses of proteolytic enzymes" from *Topics in Enzyme and Fermentation Biotechnology.* Chichester, England: Ellis Horwood Ltd., 1980, p. 25.
[2] *Primer on the Rheumatic Diseases.* Ninth Edition. Atlanta, GA: Arthritis Foundation, 1988, p. 83.
[3] Svartz, D. "The primary cause of rheumatoid arthritis is an infection – the infectious agent exists in milk." *Acta Med. Scand.* 1972; 192:231-239.
[4] Kloppenburg, M. "Minocycline in active rheumatoid arthritis."*Arthritis and Rheumatism.* 1994; 37:629-636.
[5] From personal correspondence between Dr. Bellew and Dr. Hemwall, mid-1970s.
[6] Rooney, P. "A short review of the relationship between intestinal permeability and inflammatory joint disease." *Clinical and Experimental Rheumatology.* 1990; 8:75-83.
[7] Galland, L. "Leaky gut syndromes: breaking the vicious cycle." *Townsend Letter for*

Doctors. 1995; August/September: pp. 62-68.

[8]   Crissinger, K. "Pathophysiology of gastrointestinal mucosal permeability." *Journal of Internal Medicine, Supplement*. 1990; 732:145-154.

[9]   Jenkins, R. "Increased intestinal permeability in patients with rheumatoid arthritis: a side effect of oral nonsteroidal anti-inflammatory drug therapy?" *British Journal of Rheumatology*. 1987; 26:103-107.

[10]   Bjarnason, I. "Importance of local versus systemic effects of nonsteroidal anti-inflammatory drugs in increasing small intestinal permeability in man." *Gut*. 1991; 32:275-277.

[11]   Crayhoun, R. *Nutrition Made Simple*. New York, NY: M. Evans and Company, Inc., 1994, pp. 19-25.

[12]   Lorschider, F. "Mercury exposure from 'silver tooth' fillings: emerging evidence questions a traditional dental paradigm." *The FASEB Journal*. 1995; 9:504-508.

[13]   Goyer, R. "Nutrition and metal toxicity." *American Journal of Clinical Nutrition*. 1995; 61:646S-650S.

[14]   McCarthy, G. "Dietary fish oil and rheumatic diseases." *Seminars in Arthritis and Rheumatism*. 1992; 21:368-375.

[15]   Ibid.

[16]   Simopoulos, A. "Omega-3 fatty acids in health and disease and in growth and development." American Journal of Clinical Nutrition. 1991; 54:438-463.

CHAPTER 15
Prolo Your RSD, SCI, and Other Neurological Pain Away

[1]   Merskey, H., ed. "International Association for the Study of Pain (ISAP): subcomittee on taxonomy, classification of chronic pain, description of pain terms." *Pain*. 1986; 3 (supp).

[2]   Mandel, S. "Sympathetic dystrophies." *Postgraduate Medicine*. 1990; 87:213-218.

[3]   Ibid.

[4]   Shumacker, H. "A personal overview of causalgia and other reflex dystrophies." *Annals of Surgery*. 1985; 201:278-289.

[5]   Schutzer, S. "The treatment of reflex sympathetic dystrophy syndrome." *The Journal of Bone and Joint Surgery*. 1984; 66A:625-628.

[6]   Shelton, R. "Reflex sympathetic dystrophy: a review." *Journal of the American Academy of Dermatology*. 1990; 22:513-519.

[7]   Langenskiold, A. "Osteoarthritis of the knee in the rabbit produced by immobilization: attempts to achieve a reproducible model for studies on pathogenesis and therapy." *Acta. Orthop. Scand*. 1979; 50:1.

[8]   Videman, T. "Connective tissue and immobilization." *Clinical Orthopaedics and Related Research*. 1987; 221:26-32.

[9]   Videman, T. "Experimental osteoarthritis in the rabbit: comparison of different periods of repeated immobilization." *Acta. Orthop. Scand*. 1982; 53:339.

[10]   Enneking, W. "The intra articular effects of immobilization on the human knee." *Journal of Bone and Joint Surgery*. 1972; 54:973-985.

[11]   Kottke, F., ed. *Krusen's Handbook of Physical Medicine and Rehabilitation*. Fourth Edition. Philadelphia, PA: W.B. Saunders, 1990, pp. 1122-1127.

[12]   Abramson, A. "Influence of weight-bearing and muscle contraction on disuse osteoporosis."

Archives of Physical Medicine and Rehabilitation. 1961; March:147-152.

[13]   Korr, I. "Effects of experimental myofascial insults on cutaneous patterns of sympathetic activity in man." *Journal of Neural Transmission*. 1962; 23:330-355.

[14]   Korr, I. "Experimental alterations in segmental sympathetic (sweat gland) activity through myofascial and postural disturbances." *Federal Proceedings*. 1949; 8:88.

[15]   Korr, I. "Patterns of Electrical Skin Resistance in Man." *Acta. Neuroveget (Wien)* 1958; 17:77-96.

[16]   Korr, I. "Cutaneous patterns of sympathetic activity in clinical abnormalities of the musculoskeletal system." *J. Neural Transm.* 1964; 25:589-606.

[17]   Slosberg, M. "Effects of altered afferent articular input on sensation, proprioception, muscle tone and sympathetic reflex responses." *Journal of Manipulative and Physiological Therapeutics*. 1988; 11:400-408.

[18]   Schumaker, H. "A personal overview of causalgia and other reflex dystrophies." *Annals of Surgery*. 1985; 201:278-289.

[19]   Schutzer, S. "The treatment of reflex sympathetic dystrophy syndrome." *The Journal of Bone and Joint Surgery*. 1984; 66A:625-628.

[20]   Geertzen, J. "Reflex sympathy dystrophy: early treatment and psychological aspects." *Archives of Physical Medicine and Rehabilitation*. 1994; 75:442-446.

[21]   Nepomuceno, C. "Pain in patients with spinal cord injury." *Archives of Physical Medicine and Rehabilitation*. 1979; 60:605-609.

[22]   McLeod, J. "Disorders of the autonomic nervous system: part 1. pathophysiology and clinical features." *Annals of Neurology*. 1987; 21:419-426.

[23]   Erickson, R. "Autonomic hyperreflexia: pathophysiology and medical management." *Archives of Physical Medicine and Rehabilitation*. 1980; 61:431-440.

[24]   Head, H. "Autonomic bladder, excessive sweating and some reflex conditions, in gross injuries of the spinal cord." *Brain*. 1917; 46:188-263.

[25]   Korr, I. "Effects of experimental myofascial insults on cutaneous patterns of sympathetic activity in man." *Journal of Neural Transmission*. 1962; 23:330-355.

[26]   Korr, I. "Experimental alterations in segmental sympathetic (sweat gland) activity through myofascial and postural disturbances." *Federal Procedings*. 1949; 8:88.

[27]   Korr, I. *Patterns of Electrical Skin Resistance in Man*. Acta. Neuroveget (Wien) 1958; 17:77-96.

[28]   Korr, I. "Cutaneous patterns of sympathetic activity in clinical abnormalities of the musculoskeletal system." *J. Neural Transm.* 1964; 25:589-606.

[29]   Traycoff, R. "Sacrococcygeal pain syndromes: diagnosis and treatment." *Orthopedics*. 1989; 12:1373-1377.

[30]   Ibid.

[31]   Hackett, G. "Prolotherapy for sciatica from weak pelvic ligaments and bone dystrophy." *Clinical Medicine*. 1961; p. 8.

[32]   Leijon, G. "Central post-stroke pain – a controlled trial of amitriptyline and carbamazepine." *Pain*. 1989; 36:27-36.

[33]   Leijon, G. "Central post-stroke pain – neurological symptoms and pain characteristics." *Pain*. 1989; 36:13-15.

[34]   Kiel, G. So-called initial description of phantom pain by Ambroise Pare. "Chose digne

d'admiration et quasi incredible": the "douleur es parties mortes et amputees." *Fortschr. Med.* 1990; 108:62-6.

[35] Davis, R. "Phantom sensation, phantom pain, and stump pain." *Archives of Physical Medicine and Rehabilitation.* 1993; 74:79-91.

CHAPTER 16
Prolo Your Unusual Pains Away

[1]   Mengert, W. "Referred pelvic pain." *Southern Medical Journal.* 1943; 36:256-263.

[2]   Pitikin, H. "Sacrarthrogenetic Telagia, Part Two: a study of referred pain." *Journal of Bone and Joint Surgery.* 1936; 18:365-374.

[3]   DeLisa, J. *Rehabilitation Medicine.* Philadelphia, PA: J.B. Lippincott, 1988.

[4]   Browner, B. *Skeletal Trauma.* Philadelphia, PA:W.B. Saunders Company, 1992.

[5]   Hollinshead, W. *Functional Anatomy of the Limbs and Back.* Philadelphia, PA: W.B. Saunders Company, 1981.

[6]   Taddeini, L. "Pain syndromes associated with cancer." *Postgraduate Medicine.* 1984; 75:101-108.

[7]   Laing, A. "Strontium - 89 chloride for pain palliation in prostatic skeletal malignancy." *The British Journal of Radiology.* 1991; 64:816-822.

[8]   Kirvela, O. "Treatment of painful neuromas with neurolytic blockade." *Pain.* 1990; 41:161-165.

[9]   Nidorf, D. "Proctalgia fugax." *American Family Physician.* 1995; 52:2238-2240.

[10] Ger, G. "Evaluation and treatment of chronic intractable rectal pain - a frustrating endeavor." *Diseases of the Colon and Rectum.* 1993; 36:139-145.

[11] Nidorf, D. "Proctalgia fugax." American Family Physician. 1995; 52:2238-2240.

[12] Ger, G. "Evaluation and treatment of chronic intractable rectal pain – a frustrating endeavor." *Diseases of the Colon and Rectum.* 1993; 36:139-145.

[13] Babb, R. "Proctalgia fugax." *Postgraduate Medicine.* 1996; 99:263-264.

[14] Morris, L. "Use of high voltage pulsed galvanic stimulation for patients with levator ani syndrome." *Physical Therapy.* 1987; 67:1522-1525.

[15] Tietze, A. "Uber eine eigenartige hafung ion fallen mit dystrophie der rippenknorpel." *Berl. Klin. Wchnschr.* 1921: 58:829.

[16] Rawlings, M. "The 'rib syndrome.'" *Diseases of the Chest.* 1962; 41:432-441.

[17] Davies-Colley, R. "Slipping rib." *The New England Journal of Medicine.* 296:432-433.

[18] McBeath, A. "The rib-tip syndrome." *The Journal of Bone and Joint Surgery.* 1975; 57A:795-797.

[19] Holmes, J. "A study of the slipping-rib cartilage syndrome." *The New England Journal of Medicine.* 1941; 224:928-932.

[20] Hirschberg, G. "Medical management of iliocostal pain." *Geriatrics.* 1992; 47:62-67.

[21] Ibid.

CHAPTER 17
Prolo Your Sports Injuries Away

[1]   Peterson, L. *Sports Injuries: Their Prevention and Treatment.* Chicago, IL: Year Book Medical, 1986, pp.18-63.

CHAPTER 18
Prolo Your Animal's Pain Away

[1] Smith, G. "Coxofemoral joint laxity from distraction radiography and its contemporaneous and prospective correlation with laxity, subjective score and evidence of degenerative joint disease from conventional hip-extended radiography in dogs." *American Journal of Veterinary Research*. 1993; 54:1021-1042.

[2] Fubini, S. "Effect of intramuscularly administered polysulfated glycosaminoglycan on articular cartilage from equine joints injected with methylprednisolone acetate." *American Journal of Veterinary Research*. 1993; 54:1359-1364.

[3] Chunekamrai, S. "Changes in articular cartilage after intra-articular injections of methylprednisolone acetate in horses." *American Journal of Veterinary Research*. 1989; 50:1733-1741.

[4] Trotter, G. "Effects of intra-articular administration of methylprednisolone acetate on normal equine articular cartilage." *American Journal of Veterinary Research*. 1991; 52:83-87.

[5] Shoemaker, S. "Effects of intra-articular administration of acetate on normal articular cartilage and on healing of experimentally induced osteochondral defects in horses." *American Journal of Veterinary Research*. 1992; 53:1446-1453.

[6] Megher, D. "The effects of intra-articular corticosteroids and continued training on carpal chip fractures of horses, in proceedings." *American Association of Equine Practice*. 1970; 16:405-412.

[7] From a conversation with Shaun Fauley, D.V.M., in May 1997.

[8] Chunekamrai, S. "Changes in articular cartilage after intra-articular injections of methylprednisolone acetate in horses." *American Journal of Veterinary Research*. 1989; 50:1733-1741.

[9] Pool, R. "Corticosteroid therapy in common joint and tendon injuries of the horse: effect on joints." *Proceedings of the American Association of Equine Practice*. 1980; 26:397-406.

[10] From personal correspondence between the author and Michael Herron, D.V.M.

[11] Ibid.

EPILOGUE

[1] The Holy Bible, New International Version, 2 Timothy 4:7-8.

APPENDIX A
Nutrition and Chronic Pain

[1] Reams, C. *Choose Life or Death*. Fifth Edition. Tampa, FL: Holistic Laboratories, 1990, pp. 80-85.

[2] D'Adamo, Peter. *Eat Right for Your Type*. New York, NY: G.P. Putnam's Sons, 1996.

[3] Wiley, R. *Biobalance*. Tacoma, WA: Life Sciences Press, 1989, pp. 7-18.

APPENDIX B
Neural Therapy

[1] Klinghardt, D. "Neural Therapy." *Townsend Letter for Doctors and Patients*. July 1995; pp. 96-98.

[2] Dosch, P. *Facts about Neural Therapy*. First English Edition. Heidelberg, Germany: Haug Publishers, 1985, pp. 25-30.

[3] Dosch, P. *Manual of Neural Therapy*. First English Edition. Heidelberg, Germany: Haug

Publishers, 1984, pp. 74-77.

[4] Ibid.

[5] Dosch, P. *Illustrated Atlas of the Techniques of Neural Therapy with Local Anesthetics*. First English Edition. Heidelberg, Germany: Haug Publishers, 1985.

APPENDIX F
Insurance Reimbursement Letters

[1] Capen, Karen. "Courts, licensing bodies turning their attention to alternative therapies." *Canadian Medical Associates Journal*. 1996; 156(9):1307-1308.

[2] Joel M. Greene vs. Uniform Medical Plan, June 8, 1992.

APPENDIX G
Beulah Land Natural Medicine Clinic

[1] The Holy Bible, New International Version, Revelation 21:27.

[2] The Holy Bible, New International Version, Matthew 4:23.

INDEX

A

Adhesive capsulitis, 104, 108

American Medical Association, 23, 53, 215-217

Journal of the, 23, 26, 79

Ankle pain, 135, 136, 166

Anti-inflammatory drugs, use of, 20, 21, 32, 39, 50, 62, 63, 68, 124, 127, 151-154, 156, 158, 159, 162, 192

Arachnoiditis
diagnosis of, 80, 83
pain, 81, 83
treatment of, 81

Arthritis, 31, 33, 63, 149
and NSAID use, 63
back, 77
hands, 114, 155
hips, 75
in animals, 196, 197
inflammatory, 153-156, 158, 159
knee, 122-124, 126, 127, 129
Natural Medicine approach, 154, 159, 209
of the lumbar spine, 77
Osteo, 56, 75, 114, 124, 146, 149, 150, 158, 159, 162
pain of, 149, 152, 153, 159
Rheumatoid, 20, 153-159, 206
shoulder, 107
treatment of, 77, 128, 150-153, 159

Autonomic nervous system, 90, 164, 166, 171, 205-207

B

Back pain, 23, 34, 38, 39, 42, 47, 71, 75-78, 80 81, 85, 118, 154, 181, 215

in the low, 23, 44, 48, 61, 72-76, 79, 80, 115, 118, 176, 177, 189, 206
in the mid-upper, 83, 186, 187
treatment of, 23, 32, 34, 38, 42, 44, 47, 48, 71-79, 85, 176, 181, 189

Barré-Lieou Syndrome
diagnosis of, 91, 95
symptoms of, 89-92, 95, 96
treatment of, 91, 95, 100

Beulah Land Natural Medicine Clinic, 10, 225, 226

Bone pain from cancer, 180, 181, 189

Bunions, 134, 135, 139

Buttock pain, 181

C

CAT Scan, 31, 71, 80, 81

Carpal Tunnel Syndrome, 111

Chicago Medical Society, 52, 53, 217

Chiropractic care/manipulation, 40, 54, 61, 75, 76, 93, 142, 191, 226

Coccygodynia, 167-169, 173, 183, 189

Cubital Tunnel Syndrome, 112

D

Degenerated discs, 73, 77-88

Depression, 66, 141, 144, 184

Diet (also see nutrition), 156, 157

Dizziness, 89, 91, 96, 99, 100, 205

E

Eagle Syndrome, 98, 99

Ehlers-Danlos Syndrome, 146

Elbow pain, 36, 110-112

Ernest Syndrome, 98, 99, 100

If you would like to become a patient, receive additional information, or would like Dr. Hauser to speak at a function, please contact him at:

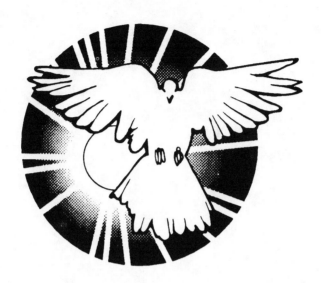

Caring Medical and Rehabilitation Services, S.C.
715 Lake St., Suite 600
Oak Park, IL 60301
(708) 848-7789
(708) 848-7763 fax
Web Site: www.caringmedical.com
E-mail: drhauser@caringmedical.com

Ross A. Hauser, M.D.
Marion A. Hauser, M.S., R.D.

The Care Of The Patient Begins With Caring

If you would like to order additional copies of this book, please call 1-800-RX-PROLO